your diet Questions answered

judith wills

Illustrations
by Nicky Dupays

quadrille

This edition published in 2006 by
Quadrille Publishing Limited,
Alhambra House,
27-31 Charing Cross Road,
London WC2H OLS

Based on material originally published
in *The Diet Bible*

EDITORIAL DIRECTOR: Jane O'Shea
CREATIVE DIRECTOR: Helen Lewis
EDITOR & PROJECT MANAGER: Lewis Esson
DESIGN: Sue Storey
PRODUCTION: Ruth Deary

Text © Judith Wills 2002 & 2006
Illustrations © Nicky Dupays 2006
Edited text, design & layout
© Quadrille Publishing Ltd 2006

ISBN-13: 978 184400 267 2
ISBN-10: 978 184400 267 5

Printed and bound in Singapore

contents and question list

You & your body 10

1 What is the difference between surplus weight and surplus fat?

2 What is the mechanism that controls body weight?

3 Does metabolic rate vary from person to person?

4 Do psychological or emotional or factors affect how I metabolize food?

5 Can I do anything to increase metabolic rate?

6 Are there foods/drinks that increase metabolism?

7 What supplements can I take to speed up my metabolism?

8 Does how or when I eat affect my metabolism?

9 Can illness affect my metabolism?

10 Is it true our weight has a natural 'set point'?

11 Is weight fluctuation throughout life normal?

12 Could my weight be due to faulty genes?

13 Could my weight problem be due to 'sluggish glands'?

14 Are there any other influences on body weight?

15 What does 'the energy equation' mean?

16 If I eat more calories than I use up, how quickly will I put on weight?

17 Can I put on weight without eating more?

18 Why do I never lose weight even though I hardly eat a thing?

19 Why do some people eat more and stay slim?

20 What causes a big appetite?

21 Why is weight easier to gain than lose?

22 What exactly is wrong with being overweight?

23 As you age is weight gain natural/desirable?

24 How are normal weight and overweight defined?

25 Is there a quick way to tell if I'm overweight?

26 What is Body Mass Index (BMI)?

27 What is 'body-fat percentage'?

28 Can dieting slow my metabolic rate?

29 Can dieting make us fat?

30 Will percentage body fat increase each time I diet?

31 Can I lose weight without dieting?

32 What's the best way to lose weight?

33 Are there operations to make me lose weight?

34 Is it a good idea to take slimming pills?

35 Why do so many people put weight back on after they've dieted?

36 How can I avoid regaining weight I've lost?

37 What factors affect my body shape?

38 I am female, with bulky arm and leg muscles. How can I get rid of them?

39 Can I choose where I lose fat via exercise?

40 How can I best work with my body shape?

41 I've slimmed, but hate my flabby bum. Any ideas?

42 Are there any instant ways of changing shape?

43 How can posture help?

44 Is a pear shape the hardest shape to change?

45 Can I spot-reduce my hips and thighs by dieting?

46 Is it true overweight mostly on the lower half of the body is quite healthy?

47 What is an apple shape and why is it unhealthy?

48 Can I lose my big tum and flabby waist without my legs getting thinner?

49 What's the best way to get a firm, flat stomach?

50 My bust is too big – can I reduce it by diet and exercise without losing off the rest of my body?

51 My face is fat and yet I'm slim – what can I do?

52 I have a month to get in shape before my holiday – what can I achieve?

53 Do you recommend a salon wrap or similar to lose weight in a hurry?

54 Now I'm slimmer, how can I exercise away skin left from when very fat?

55 What is the best exercise for making myself look taller and slimmer?

You and your food 82

56 What are calories?

57 In what types of food are calories found?

58 What happens to food in the body?

59 What happens in my body if I don't eat?

60 What happens if I eat more than I need?

61 What types of calories put on most weight?

62 Do carbohydrate foods encourage weight gain?

63 Is sugar so bad?

64 Should I use artificial sweeteners?

65 Can a high-carb, high-fibre diet help weight loss?

66 What is the Glycaemic Index?

67 What foods are best for controlling hunger?

68 How do I avoid feeling weak/tired/dizzy on a diet?

69 Do I need to feel pangs of hunger to lose weight?

70 Does a high-protein diet have special benefits?

71 Does fat make you fat?

72 What are the different types of fat?

73 Is a low-fat diet always the best way to slim?

74 What is food combining?

75 Is eating nothing but raw food a good idea?

76 Does a diet high in fruit and veg help weight loss?

77 Is regular snacking between meals a good idea?

78 How many meals a day is best for weight loss?

79 How important is breakfast in a good slimming campaign?

80 Does food eaten late convert straight to body fat while you sleep?

81 What are the best drinks on a slimming diet?

82 How do I pick the right diet?

83 Is there such as thing as 'the perfect diet'?

84 What are the most popular diets?

85 How many calories do you need to reduce to daily to lose weight?

86 What is a crash diet?

87 Are crash diets really such a bad idea?

88 Is fasting a good idea for weight loss?

89 What's the least calories I can eat to slim healthily long-term?

90 What are the pros/cons of very-low-cal, liquid diets?

91 Can you block calories in food so they're unabsorbed?

92 Is it true there are foods with 'negative calories'?

93 Can I slim without drastic diet changes?

94 What's the most reliable and easy way to slim and maintain weight?

95 What is the 'traffic light guide' to eating?

96 Is it best to avoid dairy produce when slimming?

97 Could a food allergy be causing my inability to lose weight?

98 Does avoiding wheat products help you to lose weight?

99 Are there disadvantages to diets restricted to just a few types of food?

100 I enjoy fast food. Is it really necessary to cut these out to lose weight?

101 How do the fat and calorie content of various fast foods compare?

102 I love chocolate – can I eat it as part of a diet?

103 I have a sweet tooth and can't live without desserts – suggestions?

104 I love cheese - can my diet cope with its calories?

105 What are the best (quick and easy) cooking methods for slimmers?

106 What are the best tips for reducing calories in my food painlessly?

You and your life 152

107 I should lose weight – but can't get motivated?

108 I've lost weight and it returns – why bother?

109 Everyone says diets don't work – why bother?

110 Everyone says I look fine as I am – so why slim?

111 I'd like to lose weight but my family don't want me to – what do I do?

112 Ours is a food-dominated society – how do I slim against the odds?

113 Food is my main pleasure – why should I deny myself?

114 Aren't overweight people just greedy/lazy?

115 Is there an answer to diet food being boring?

116 What are the best tips for delicious dieting?

117 Is there a way to beat comfort eating on carbs?

118 How do I stop eating when bored?

119 I eat when angry and/or frustrated – any ideas?

120 I've no willpower, so can't diet – any tips?

121 Is my need for food hunger or habit?

122 What's the difference between greed and hunger?

123 I am a chocoholic. Can chocolate be addictive?

124 I'm disorganized – how do I reduce calories?

125 I've always existed on junk food. How can I slim?

126 I can't seem to turn down food, even when not hungry – any ideas?

127 I can easily go all day with virtually no food, but in the evening I crave food. What am I doing wrong?

128 Is there an 'Alcoholics Anonymous' for the overweight?

129 I'm overweight, but a feminist – isn't dieting female submission?

130 Are there alternative remedies or natural treatments for overeating?

131 Are there slimming equivalents of one-to-one life coaches?

132 Can you recommend books to help me slim?

133 How do I retrain my tastebuds to healthy food?

134 What are eating disorders, who gets them and why?

135 What are the signs of anorexia?

136 Will rigorous dieting make me likely to suffer from anorexia?

137 How do I recognize someone with bulimia?

138 I'm told I'm too thin but feel fat. Should I diet?

139 I make myself sick for weight loss. Is this OK?

140 I often eat masses. Do I have a disorder?

141 Is 'night bingeing' an eating disorder?

142 How can I slim if I'm too busy to diet?

143 I sleep 4 hours a night – do I burn more calories?

144 Does mental activity burn calories?

145 Does stress burn calories?

146 Does smoking keep you slim?

147 I've given up smoking – is weight gain inevitable?

148 Any ideas for quick, easy, non-fattening tasty suppers for 1 or 2?

149 Is it OK to diet on convenience foods?

150 Is there such a thing as a non-fattening takeaway or fast-food meal, for my main meal?

151 I work night shifts – is there a diet for me?

152 I haven't time for breakfast and have my main meal late in the evening. Can this cause weight gain?

153 I'm ravenous when I get home from work. How do I stop myself snacking?

154 How do I resist the snacks trolley at work?

155 I travel a lot and eat at pubs and cafés. What can I do to slim?

156 Is skipping lunch a good way to slim?

157 Our cafeteria majors on pies, chips, sausage, etc. What's the best bet?

158 I travel a lot and am entertained in homes and restaurants. How do I avoid weight gain?

159 Can you give me ideas for healthy low-fat lunch-box meals?

160 Are there tempting non-fattening snacks?

161 I'm often entertained in restaurants, which has made me fat. What do I do?

162 I often stay in hotels – any advice on their menus?

163 I am often invited to dinner in people's homes. How do I eat fewer calories without causing offence?

164 Surely the best way to eat out and stay slim is to say 'no' to carbs?

165 Eating out, should I go for starter and main course or main course and dessert?

166 Which desserts are least calorific?

167 I eat out a lot, so don't want the restriction of a 'set diet'. Any guidelines?

168 I eat sensibly but drink a bottle of wine nightly. Has this caused my weight gain?

169 What are your tips for cutting down on alcohol? .

170 I'm tempted to nibble while cooking; any tips?

171 How can I stop eating the food I buy for kid's lunch boxes – cakes, etc?

172 I've only £15/week to spend on food. Any ideas?

173 I'm a student living in a bedsit – what can I eat that's cheap but slimming?

174 I need a healthy non-fattening main meal of the day at about £1/head for 4. Can you advise?

175 Is it OK to cut out meat and dairy produce to save calories?

176 Can a vegetarian diet give me all the nutrients I need?

You and your health and fitness 238

177 What are the links between weight and health?

178 If I put on weight, how soon will it begin to affect my health?

179 How overweight do you have to be before you get health problems?

180 Does being overweight shorten life span?

181 I'm overweight but feel healthy, should I worry?

182 If I've been fat for a long time, can I reverse ill health if I lose weight?

183 What's the healthiest slimming diet in the world?

184 Are all slimming diets healthy?

185 Are all healthy diets slimming?

186 Are there healthy fats that can help weight loss?

187 If crash dieting isn't healthy, why has a doctor put my very overweight husband on a very-low-calorie liquid diet?

188 Is yo-yo dieting bad and can I lose weight after years of yo-yoing?

189 What is 'low blood sugar' and why do dieters apparently often get it?

190 Can you recommend a slimming diet for diabetics?

191 What are the health advantages of a detox diet?

192 Will a detox diet help me to lose weight?

193 What's the best slimming diet for someone with high blood pressure?

194 What's the best diet for someone with arthritis?

195 What causes an apple shape, why is it unhealthy and how can I beat it?

196 Why does being overweight raise the risk of heart trouble?

197 What is the ideal weight and diet for a healthy heart?

198 Should I go to the doctor for help in dieting?

199 Can you be overweight and yet fit?

200 How does fitness affect weight?

201 In what ways does being fit affect health?

202 How does exercise help you diet when it increases appetite?

203 I hate exercise – what's the best calorie-burning exercise for me?

204 What exactly is aerobic exercise?

205 How often do I have to exercise in order to lose weight?

206 How long do I have to exercise for at a time to lose weight?

207 How much weight can I lose through exercise?

208 Is the best exercise for slimming 'short and sharp' or 'long and slow'?

209 I exercise 40 minutes every day by walking my child to school, but I don't lose weight. Why?

210 What low-cost exercise can help lose weight?

211 What's the best calorie-burning programme for an unfit beginner?

212 I can spare 10 minutes a day and am reasonably fit. Which exercise will burn up the most calories in that time?

213 Can you recommend home exercise equipment to help burn calories?

214 What's the best all-round programme to keep fit and lose weight?

215 Which exercise, apart from weight training, is good for muscles?

216 When exercising, what's the difference between burning calories and burning fat?

217 Does everybody burn calories at the same rate during exercise?

218 Which is the best exercise – walking, running or swimming?

219 How much exercise is too much?

220 Which aerobic exercise is good for tone?

221 What's the best exercise for flattening tums?

222 What are my 'training zone' and my 'maximum heart rate'?

223 What's the best time to exercise in order to burn the most fat?

224 Which is best for weight control – weight training or aerobic exercise?

225 How does strength training help me to lose weight?

226 Does muscle turn into fat when you stop exercise?

227 Will isometrics help me lose weight?

228 Can you get fit and slim through gentle exercise, such as yoga?

229 How much weight can I lose if I join the gym?

230 Is there any type of exercise I should avoid if I am very fat?

231 Can I exercise on an empty stomach?

232 When is it unwise to exercise?

You and your special needs 306
For women only 308

233 However hard I try to lose weight, before every period I put on 5 pounds. How can I avoid this?

234 I get depressed before my period, and this makes me comfort eat. What can I do?

235 Before my period, I crave sweet foods, particularly chocolate. What can I do about it?

236 I feel hungrier and eat more in the few days before my period. Is there a cause and cure?

237 At period time I crave carbs, particularly bread. Why is this?

238 Before every period, I swell up due to fluid retention, which makes me feel fat and miserable. What can I do about it?

239 Why do women naturally have much more body fat than men?

240 Does sex burn off lots of calories?

241 What is cellulite and is it caused by toxins?

242 Why don't men get cellulite?

243 Why do even slim women get cellulite?

244 How can I get rid of cellulite?

245 I'd like to get pregnant, but I'm very overweight. Does this matter?

246 Should I eat for two when pregnant?

247 What's the best way to lose weight during pregnancy?

248 I'm putting on weight too fast during this pregnancy; any advice?

249 What is the right amount of weight to gain during pregnancy?

250 If an average baby weighs about 8lb, can't I just put on 8lb so when baby is born I will be my correct weight?

251 If I crave foods when pregnant does my body need their nutrients?

252 Is plenty of exercise the best way to keep weight down during pregnancy or should I just put my feet up?

253 When my baby is born what's the best way to get my figure back and how soon can I exercise?

254 What is the best exercise to get my stomach back into shape after the birth?

255 I need to lose weight but I'm breast-feeding. How can I slim safely?

256 If not breast-feeding, what calorie intake do I aim for to slim?

257 Does HRT cause weight gain?

258 Is weight gain inevitable for a woman during/after menopause?

259 Is mid-life weight gain for a woman healthy?

260 Is it possible to lose weight while going through the menopause and on HRT?

261 My body seems to have slowed down since the menopause. What can I do?

262 Should one eat less as one gets older?

263 Is it ever too late to start a diet?

For men only 342

264 Is there a difference in diets for men and for women?

265 As alcohol helps prevent heart disease, should I carry on drinking and cut calories elsewhere?

266 I'm not overweight but I've put 4 inches on my waist. I'm 50. Is this normal – and reversible?

267 Does beer drinking really cause a 'beer belly'?

268 When I gain weight, why does it go to my belly?

269 Is a pot belly a cause for concern?

270 How do I slim my pot belly but keep the rest of my shape?

271 Can I do anything about my flabby 'breasts'?

272 Are there fat-burning exercise classes not aimed at women?

273 I dislike the gym and outdoor exercise. How do I burn calories?

274 Is there a male menopause and if so has it caused my weight gain?

For kids (and parents) only 350

275 How do I tell if my child is overweight?

276 What is the best way to prevent a child from becoming overweight?

277 Is it true you shouldn't put a child on a low-cal diet?

278 What's the best way to slim a child down?

279 Should I take my overweight child to the doctor?

280 How can I stop my child from liking junk food as it is making him fat?

281 My son has a huge appetite and is gaining weight, yet if I cut portions he gets very hungry. What can I do?

282 Is it OK to reduce fat in children's diets?

283 If my child is overweight is fat the first thing to restrict?

284 Is a high-fibre diet suitable for all children?

285 How can I avoid my child eating sweets when she starts school?

286 What's the best way with a child's high intake of sweets and chocolate – banning them or using them as occasional treats?

287 Any ideas for healthy, less fattening alternatives to sweets and crisps?

288 My boy is overweight but goes into tantrums if I don't give him what he wants. What can I do?

289 I have 3 children, but only one is overweight, causing endless problems at meal times. Any ideas?

290 Do you have main meal ideas for overweight children who only really like burgers, chips, etc?

291 My son prefers the most unhealthy/fattening items; how can I lead him to healthier choices?

292 How do I give my kids reduced-fat/calorie meals so they don't realize?

293 What's the best form of exercise for an exercise-shy child?

294 What's a good breakfast for a child who is mildly overweight?

295 Can you advise me on healthy low-cal packed lunches for my children?

296 Is there such a thing as puppy fat?

297 Is any exercise dangerous for a child?

298 How does one stop a child from getting obsessive about dieting?

299 What are the signs of anorexia or bulimia?

300 What should I do if I think my child may have an eating disorder?

Index 382

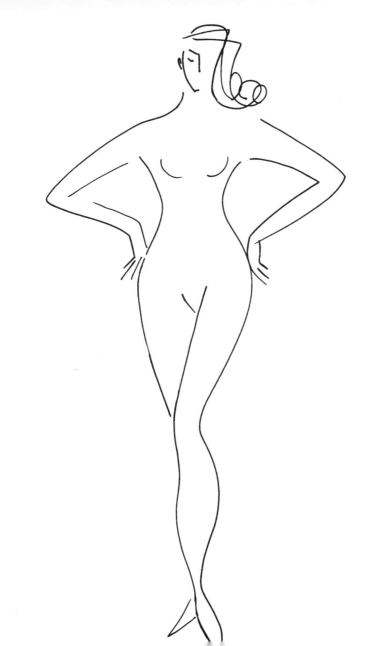

It's been estimated that 30% of females and 25% of males in the UK and 40% of females and 24% of males in the USA are trying to lose weight at any given time. We're desperate to lose weight – but nothing's working, and lack of knowledge could be the key. There are almost as many misconceptions about weight control as there are overweight people. When you're dissatisfied with your body, it's not always your weight you hate, but your shape. Maybe the big hips or bottom if you're female, or the paunch if male. It seems whatever shape we're in, we're rarely satisfied. So in this section we aim to separate fact from fiction; from metabolism to appetite, from weight assessment to the best ways to lose weight, from why you're the shape you are to what can be done to change the parts you dislike by means of diet, exercise, etc.

you and your body

When people become overweight or obese, their body-fat percentage increases, while changes in muscle and bone mass are usually relatively small. Weight increase due to altered bone mass is highly unlikely – even a 10% increase in bone mass would account for only an extra 2–3 lb (1–1.5kg) of body weight.

Muscle weighs more than fat and bone, and can also be increased quite drastically over time by means of exercise and good nutrition. So, somebody with a high muscle mass (for example, a weightlifter or field-sportsperson) could weigh much more than average, meaning that they would be overweight under the Body Mass Index classifications (see Question 26), while having no more body fat than an average person.

In this case, a waist test or 10-second test (see Question 25) or a body fat monitoring test (using special callipers or electronic body fat monitors) is a much more reliable indication of body fat; and if body fat percentage turns out to be low, then there is no need to lose weight. It is, indeed, highly unlikely that your

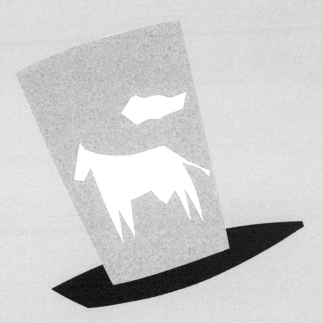

surplus weight can be accounted for by increased muscle mass without you knowing about it – and a look in the mirror will obviously show muscle definition and tone, not flab.

Occasionally, fluid retention can account for surplus weight. Several conditions (such as premenstrual syndrome in women) and diseases (such as heart disease) can mean that the body retains more fluid than usual. This is often apparent (e.g. a swollen face, stomach, ankles). If you feel that it may be fluid, you should see your doctor. For 99% of us, however, surplus weight usually equals surplus fat.

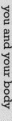

Q2

What is the basic mechanism that controls my body weight?

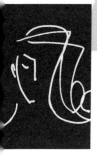

Your weight – particularly body fat – reflects the balance between your energy intake and expenditure. Intake is everything you eat or drink containing calories and expenditure is the calories your body burns up for fuel.

There are three categories of energy expenditure. The first is your basal metabolic rate (BMR) or calories you burn up just existing – i.e. doing absolutely nothing. On average, this accounts for roughly 60% of energy used. The second is the energy used in activity – moving, talking, etc. – which accounts for an average of 30% of calories used. Lastly is dietary thermogenesis or 'meal-induced heat production', the calories used in eating and digesting food, accounting for 10% of calories used.

If energy input and output balance, our weight remains stable. If input is higher, then the surplus energy is stored as body fat. If output is higher than input, fat stores are converted back into energy and, over time, we lose weight. The amount of your energy output over a period of time is known as your metabolic rate.

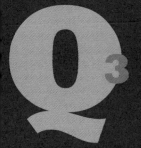

Q₃

Does the metabolic rate vary from person to person and is it true that fat people have a slow metabolic rate?

A

The rate at which the body burns calories – at rest, during activity and via dietary thermogenesis (opposite) – varies considerably with gender, age, weight, fitness, body composition, the duration and intensity of activity, and the food you eat. There are also genetic, hormonal, etc. factors. The World Health Organization estimates basal metabolic rate alone can vary as much as 25% between individuals of similar weight. This is why to keep weight steady some people have to eat little and others a great deal.

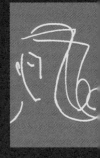

Fat people don't have a slow metabolic rate; in fact, other factors being equal, the heavier you are the higher your rate, as a heavy body uses more energy both at BMR level and to move around, fat-free mass (muscle and other tissue) also generally increases with weight, and dietary thermogenesis increases. Hence, when fat people lose lots of weight their new metabolic rate is considerably reduced. However, research has found heavy people move around less than slim people and do less demanding activity, burning fewer calories.

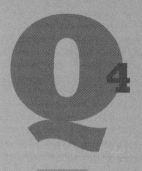

Q4

Do emotional or psychological factors affect how I metabolize food?

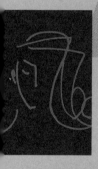

It's well known that emotional factors influence our hormones, and vice versa. For example, one well-known hormone, adrenalin (epinephrine), is released when we are frightened, anxious or excited. Adrenalin speeds up metabolic rate.

If you're a very laid-back, contented person, with little excitement in your life, you probably have fewer bursts of adrenalin (epinephrine) release and this could in theory predispose you to weight gain. All the slim and relaxed people in the world will disagree here, of course. Stress may make you more 'fidgety' and it has been shown that fidgeting can burn up many hundreds of calories in a day.

However, in the long-term, stress can also make you fat! The adrenal hormone cortisol, released when you're stressed, can increase fat storage in the abdominal area as, it seems, the deep fat in the stomach contains receptors that the cortisol prefers. Also, a surfeit of stress triggers cortisol to boost blood sugar levels (in preparation for 'fight or flight') which, if not used, are converted by insulin into fat for storage.

Can I do anything to increase my own metabolic rate?

You can alter your basal metabolic rate (BMR) by increasing your lean tissue (muscle), as muscle uses more calories than other tissue, even resting. You can be more active to burn extra calories – the average is 30%, but many sedentary people use only about 15% more calories than their BMR in activity, while 50% or more of the metabolic rate of very active people is accounted for by activity. You can also alter dietary thermogenesis by tweaking food intake. If losing weight, however, it's harder to increase metabolic rate, because you'll also naturally reduce your BMR at the same time (Question 3).

The foolproof way to increase metabolic rate is to take more regular exercise. Recent research demonstrated that high-intensity (i.e. hard!) exercise raised heart rate, metabolic rate and energy expenditure for several hours. Exercise should include aerobic work to increase calorie and fat burning plus strength work to increase lean tissue. For every extra pound of muscle, your body uses 50 or so more calories daily. A recent study found regular weight training boosts BMR by about 15%.

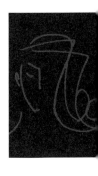

you and your body

17

Are there any foods or drinks that can increase my metabolic rate?

Protein foods have an above average dietary thermogenic effect – as we saw in Question 2, eating food produces heat, which equals calorie usage of around 10% of total energy expenditure. Eating pure protein, however, produces a higher thermogenic effect – up to 25% of such a meal's calories may be burnt due to thermogenesis. In theory, this means a diet with high levels of protein would result in considerable speeding of the metabolism. However, this isn't a good idea, as a high-protein diet can stress the kidneys and liver, is linked with loss of bone calcium and possibly higher blood pressure. In addition, such a diet is not balanced and nutrients in other food groups may be in shortfall.

Some protein foods – particularly red meat and dairy produce – contain a fatty acid called conjugated linoleic acid (CLA), which has been shown to increase lean tissue and may therefore increase metabolic rate. Eggs contain the amino acid leucine, which helps the body burn fat and control hunger, while a research study has shown that obese people who regularly ate yogurt as part of a low-calorie diet lost 61% more fat than people on a normal low-calorie diet. Fresh nuts, like almonds, also seem to have a metabolism-boosting effect according to some research, possibly because of their omega oils.

Spices, particularly chilli, can raise metabolic rate by up to 50% for up to three hours, probably due to heart rate increase. Spices are healthy in other ways, so this is one metabolism-boosting trick you can use without guilt.

Caffeine-containing drinks increase the metabolism by arousing the nervous system's flight response and levels of adrenalin (epinephrine), increasing heart rate and 'fidget factor'. Caffeine equivalent to 2.5 cups of coffee can also increase endurance during moderate exercise. Coffee and colas are two of the drinks highest in caffeine. However, more than three or four cups of high-caffeine coffee a day isn't recommended, because of possible adverse effects on health. Caffeine is also found in chocolate, tea and a range of manufactured drinks.

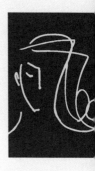

Interestingly, green tea also appears to stimulate the metabolism without increasing heart rate. A study found people who took extract of green tea burned more calories than people who didn't. Its phytochemical flavonoids seem to speed the process of fat oxidation.

If you have an iodine deficiency, which may result in poor thyroid functioning, production of the hormone thyroxine may be low. This may lower metabolic rate, and a diet rich in sea greens (such as dulse, kombu or wakame), seafood and milk can raise iodine levels and improve thyroid function and metabolism. If your thyroid function is normal, however, these foods won't help.

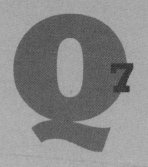

CLA capsules (see the previous question) appear to increase the metabolic rate by increasing lean tissue. As far as we know, they are perfectly safe to take although quite expensive.

If your levels of body iodine are low, your thyroid function may be impaired, which can, in turn, reduce metabolic rate, and you may benefit from iodine-rich supplements such as kelp (or there are several multi-ingredient, so-called thyroid-boosting, supplements available, which may include l-tyrosine, an amino acid that helps produce thyroxine). If you are not deficient, however, these supplements won't boost thyroid function, and dosing yourself without knowing whether or not you are deficient is probably unwise, as overdosing can be toxic and can actually suppress thyroid function (see Question 13 for more on the thyroid).

Supplements of DHEA (dehydroepiandrosterone), a naturally occurring steroid hormone, are said, among other things, to increase lean tissue and reduce body fat; however, you should be cautious about taking these.

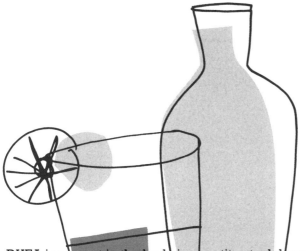

DHEA is present in the body in quantity at adolescence, and levels diminish over time after the age of 30. There have been concerns over its long-term safety and for many people benefits may be small or non-existent, unless a blood test shows you are deficient. In the UK, it is available on prescription only, but in the USA it is sold as a food supplement.

One recent trial found that supplements of a Chinese herbal preparation, Ma Huang (containing a natural form of the stimulant ephedrine), worked to help volunteers lose weight without strict dieting and the researchers concluded that this herbal supplement had a less adverse effect on the blood pressure than the new prescription slimming drug sibutramine (Reductil).

Other supplements used as aids to slimming include amino acids, such as L-carnitine, caffeine (including guarana), chromium, co-enzyme Q10 and creatine.

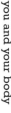

you and your body

Does how or when – rather than what – I eat affect my metabolism?

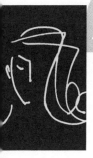

There is support for the theory that eating small regular meals is a better way to burn calories than, say, one meal a day. Levels of hormones controlling metabolic rate drop within hours of eating. Also, the thermogenic effect of dividing calorie intake over several meals may be higher.

Studies found infrequent meal patterns are associated with obesity and obese people had a better chance of losing weight by eating little and often, as hunger is better controlled and there's less inclination to binge.

Eating in the hours after brisk exercise may encourage metabolism of food rather than storing it as fat, as metabolic rate is higher. Similarly, moderate exercise (e.g. a walk) after eating may increase thermogenic response to food and burn more calories. There's good reason to eat slowly, though; one study found obese people eat faster.

There is no convincing evidence that eating at any particular time speeds metabolism. A large study found those who had most food late in the day consumed more calories, so weight gain associated with evening eating is likely to be to do with calories consumed.

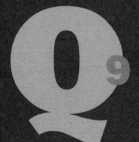

Q9

Can illness affect my metabolism?

A Diseases of the metabolism-controlling thyroid and/or pituitary gland, such as hypothyroidism and thyroiditis, can cause weight gain. Tumours of the adrenal or pituitary glands may produce Cushing's disease, causing facial and abdominal weight gain. Corticosteroids given to treat many medical conditions, including rheumatoid arthritis, may also cause Cushing's.

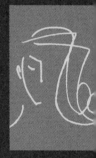

Severe depression may lower metabolic rate and some drugs (tricyclic) used to treat depression can also do so. Many types of long illness or incapacity may lower metabolic rate, as they predispose to bed rest and/or inactivity, reducing lean tissue and burning fewer calories.

Temporarily, high fever will increase metabolic rate; 10% for every degree C increase. In the later stages of cancer, rapid weight loss not due to reduced food intake is often present, possibly due to raised metabolism.

Several fairly common prescription drugs may cause weight gain, apart from those already mentioned. If you think your weight gain may be due to illness or drugs, talk to your doctor.

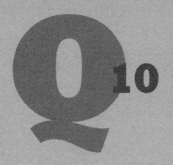

Q10

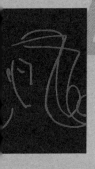

The 'set point' theory says the body has a 'natural' weight it tries to keep. For example, if your body is happy with its weight and you diet below it your body will do all it can to revert to it. This would explain why 95% of slimmers put weight on again – they've been aiming too low.

The theory falls down applied in reverse – i.e. if you pile on pounds, the body doesn't seem so keen to return to a lower weight, so most of us gain weight gradually as we age. (Theory proponents argue that the set point resets itself upwards as we age.)

Research confirms the body probably exerts a stronger defence against low calorie intake and weight loss than high intake and weight gain: i.e. it protects stored fat. Drastic restriction of calories can suppress metabolic rate by up to 45%, a mechanism thought to have evolved as a defence against starvation.

However, 'set point' theory IS still debated and, even if confirmed, the consensus is regular exercise can alter it by increasing lean tissue, raising BMR and facilitating fat breakdown.

you and your body

24

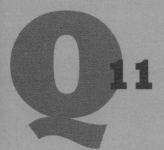

Q11 Is weight fluctuation throughout life normal?

There are not many people who stay at exactly the same weight throughout their adult lives, so yes; fluctuation is normal rather than the exception. For example, weight can be lost through illness, by loss of appetite, through reduced food intake at busy times or through periods of increased activity. Weight may increase due to other sets of circumstances, such as holidays, celebrations, etc.

Apart from these periodic – and usually short-lived – changes, which shouldn't concern you unduly, the average pattern of weight gain and loss is as follows: weight tends to be lowest during the teens and early 20s, when calorie needs are greatest, then static in the later 20s and early 30s, gradually increasing in middle age up until around 65, when many people slowly begin to lose weight again into old age. This is an average pattern – which means you don't have to follow it.

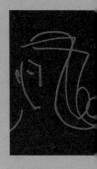

you and your body

25

The wide-ranging report on obesity published in 2000 by the World Health Organization concluded that 'while it is possible that single or multiple gene effects may cause overweight and obesity directly, and indeed do so in some individuals, this does not appear to be the case in the majority of people'.

However, the consensus of expert opinion is that your genes can have at least some influence on your susceptibility to be overweight. An overview of all the studies on the genetic influence suggests that 25–40% of cases of obesity have a hereditary factor and that intra-abdominal fat appears to have a genetic link of up to 60%. One study of twins concluded that 60% of body fat is determined by genetics. An American research study in 2003 actually identified two forms of the GAD2 gene in humans, one of which protects against obesity while the other increases appetite and hunger.

If one of your parents is overweight, you may have inherited that parent's 'fat genes'. If both are overweight, it may be you are very unlucky and they both have faulty fat genes – but it is probably more likely that, as a family, you eat too many calories and don't take enough exercise. As one US researcher remarked, 'The human gene pool cannot possibly have altered so much in the last 30 years to account for the vast rise in the incidence of obesity' and, in the words of another, 'You don't get fat in a famine.' Whatever the reasons, one estimate is that a child with two fat parents has a 70% chance of growing up obese.

Even if you have inherited a tendency to put on weight, it doesn't mean you can't lose weight or maintain a reasonable weight but that, for example, you may be more likely than someone without 'fat genes' to put on weight given the same amount of food.

A few specific examples of how your genes may influence your weight:
• By giving you a BMR lower than average.
• By giving you a high percentage of body fat and a low percentage of lean tissue, predisposing you to needing fewer calories than average for your height and weight.
• By giving you a larger-than-average appetite (see Question 20).
• By giving you a blunted thermic response to food, meaning your dietary-induced thermogenesis will be lower than average, causing a higher number of calories to be stored rather than burnt.

Research is being carried out in all these areas and it may be possible in future to reprogramme gene defects so such people don't get fat. Meanwhile, the message is that by maintaining a balance of calories in and calories out, most people can maintain a reasonable body weight.

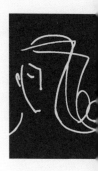

you and your body

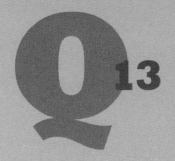

Q13 Could my weight problem be due to 'sluggish glands'?

As we've seen in the answers to Questions 7, 9 and 14, any malfunction of the thyroid glands, which help regulate metabolism, can cause weight gain if either of two hormones produced by these glands – thyroxine or T3 (triiodothyronine) – is insufficient. This is termed hypothyroidism. (Another dysfunction, hyperthyroidism, produces too much hormone and weight may then be lost due to this.)

This can come about in a variety of ways: if mild it may be corrected by increasing your intake of iodine, which is vital in the production of the thyroid hormones; if more severe, you may need artificial thyroid drugs.

If you think you have a thyroid problem (other symptoms may include cold hands and feet, feeling sluggish and lacking in energy, constipation, dry skin) you should talk to your doctor, who can arrange a blood test. If this is the problem and it is corrected, surplus weight should gradually go and your metabolic rate fairly quickly be restored to normal.

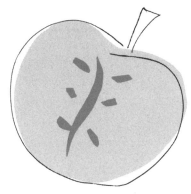

Problems with the adrenal glands may possibly also contribute to weight problems. Some specialists say that, with a permanently stressed life, these glands – which produce the stress hormones epinephrine (adrenalin) and norepinephrine (noradrenaline), and cortisol – get 'exhausted' and this can set off a chain of events that may produce weight gain. Again, you need to see your doctor if you have long-term stress and have gained weight disproportionately to the amount you eat.

By the way, interestingly, some foods seem to suppress the action of the thyroid – particularly soya beans and soya products, and also members of the brassica family including cabbage, cauliflower, spinach and Brussels sprouts.

Lastly, it is estimated that of all cases of obesity, only a maximum of 3% are actually caused by an underactive thyroid, so don't be too surprised if this isn't your problem.

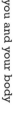

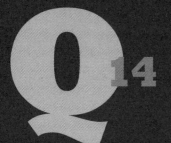

Q14

A

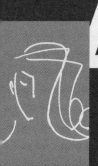

The body processes that regulate weight are many and diverse, and orchestrated by our hormones. As US obesity specialist Jules Hirsch wrote in the *British Medical Journal*, 'The balance of food intake and energy expenditure that maintains constant energy storage is determined by the metabolism of muscle, liver, pancreas and intestine. The balance is regulated by the adrenal and sex steroids as well as adipose tissue itself, which together create a complex set of signals... affecting energy dissipation and food intake. Hovering over this complex system are potent psychosocial and behavioural factors.' He concludes by remarking on the 'incredible intricacy and complexity of the system that maintains a fixed level of energy storage'.

So your answer is yes, there are other influences – and researchers are only really beginning to unravel the whole complicated system! However, you needn't worry about it too much. All you really need to know is whether or not you're managing your own energy balance successfully enough to maintain a reasonable weight.

Q15

What does 'the energy equation' mean?

The energy equation is a way of expressing how your body balances intake and expenditure of energy (calories): Change in stored energy (body weight) = energy intake – energy expenditure. Meaning:

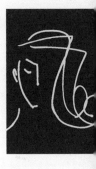

• If energy intake equals expenditure there'll be no change in stored energy (body weight).
• If intake exceeds expenditure, there'll be an increase in stored energy (weight gain): a positive energy balance.
• If expenditure exceeds intake, there'll be a decrease in stored energy (weight loss): a negative energy balance.

In theory, weight gain or loss can be measured as: 3,500 calories ingested in excess of expenditure means 1lb (450g) gain; 3,500 calories burnt in excess of intake means 1lb (450g) loss. 3,500 calories don't always equal 1lb (450g), but it's a reasonable blueprint on which all diet regimes rely.

As the body converts surplus food (fat, carbohydrate or protein) to fat, for 'stored energy' read 'fat'. Paradoxically, however, some weight lost by creating a negative energy balance is lean tissue. Water losses/gains are not accounted for in the equation, as water is calorie-free.

Q16

If I eat more calories than I use up, how quickly will I put on weight?

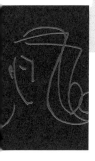

As in the previous answer, eating 3,500 calories over that needed by the body to maintain its current weight will result in a gain of 1lb (450g). If, say, you need around 2,500 calories a day to maintain your weight, and you eat 500 calories a day more than this every day for a week, without making any other changes, you will be giving your body 3,500 more calories than it needs (500 x 7 = 3,500), and you will, in theory, put on 1lb (450g).

So it all depends on how much more you eat than you need. You'd have a job putting on 1lb a day as eating an extra 3,500 calories a day is quite hard, giving the lie to people who say they put on pounds when they go out for a meal. What really happens in this case is that much of the weight gained 'overnight' is, in fact, fluid retained by a meal high in carbohydrates and sodium. Most people generally overeat only slightly and thus put on weight very gradually.

you and your body

Q17

Is it possible to put on weight without eating more?

Yes, it is. A positive energy balance (weight gain, see Question 15) can be achieved not just by increasing energy input (eating more) but also by decreasing energy output (doing less physical activity). Any active sportsperson who then gives up and puts on weight knows this only too well. For example, if you give up one hour a day of, say, walking to work, but continue to eat in the same way, you'd be expending about 200 calories a day less, i.e. 1,400 calories expenditure less a week – leading to a weight gain of about 1lb in $2\frac{1}{2}$ weeks! And they say exercise doesn't help you lose weight!

Although reduced physical activity is the main cause of weight gain other than overeating, other variables may also be at play. For example, as you get older your metabolism slows slightly, all other factors being equal, so that would cause a slow weight gain. Illness, depression, drugs and other factors may also be involved in unexplained weight gain. If you feel you're gaining weight without good reason, talk to your doctor.

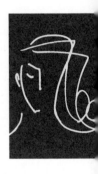

you and your body

Q18

Why do I never lose weight even though I hardly eat a thing?

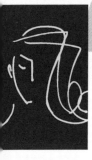

Firstly, you may already be at a reasonable weight – people come in all shapes and sizes, largely governed by genetics, and there's a wide range of weights within which you're still 'average'. If you are your 'natural' weight at, say, 10 stone, it'll be hard to slim to $8^{1}/_{2}$. So aim for a reasonable weight. Check your BMI in Question 26.

If you're overweight – not obese – it could be that your metabolic rate is low, because you don't take enough exercise and have a small proportion of lean tissue. Your rate may be genetically slower than average – another reason to aim for a reasonable weight. As we age, metabolic rate tends to slow (see Question 23) and menopause reduces it slightly.

If these don't answer your problem, it may be you're taking in more calories than you think. Most studies of slimmers, comparing actual calorie intake with reported intake, have shown underestimates of 12–25%. People underestimate portions, forget calories in drinks or foods nibbled while preparing meals, etc. Try measuring your food and keeping a food diary.

you and your body

34

Q19

Why do some people eat a lot more than me and yet stay slim?

How much you can eat without weight gain depends on metabolic rate – the rate at which you burn calories. Some people have a high rate – say, burning 3,500 cals/day (and are able to eat more without gaining weight); others a slow one – say, burning only 1,700 cals/day (and must eat less to stay slim). 200 Leeds volunteers were studied and it was found that the metabolic rate of lean people asleep is faster than fatter counterparts.

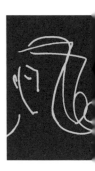

One theory is that people who gain weight easily have a blunted thermal response to eating. In some, dietary induced thermogenesis (Question 2) accounts for a rise in metabolic rate of 30% after eating, but in many fat people this is nearer 5%. Weight gain would thus be much more likely for the latter, vindicating at least some overweight people who claim they hardly eat a thing.

Also research shows many thin people who seem to eat a lot actually eat less than overweight people – preferring, say, salads and fruit. Recent research at the USA's Mayo Clinic found overweight people sit still on average for $2\frac{1}{2}$ hours longer each day than those of normal weight.

What causes a big appetite and can it be controlled?

Appetite is a basic survival mechanism, ensuring we seek sustenance to stay alive. Many experts believe a big appetite is a natural reminder of the anthropologically not-too-distant past when food wasn't easy to find. When we did, we ate all we could, not sure when there'd be more – surplus stored as fat would normally be used before the next meal. Today, food is so plentiful we never get a chance to use our stores, but this mechanism hasn't caught up.

Other factors are involved. One study on rodents showed they ate more when offered a variety of foods against a restricted range. Many of us do the same – think of fresh 'appetite' after a meal when pudding appears. Anything new also has a similar effect. You may also experience increased appetite when eating favourite foods. Habitual eating – certain things at certain times – is also often mistaken for true appetite. High levels of physical activity seem to increase appetite in lean people – to restore energy balance – but not in obese people.

In women, appetite increases during latter pregnancy and the pre-menstrual phase. Seasonal affective disorder

(SAD) may also increase appetite for carbs, which help produce the 'happy' neurotransmitter, serotonin. Scientists are just beginning to unravel the chemicals, proteins and hormones affecting appetite. For over 10 years, they've known about the hormone leptin, a product of the 'ob' obesity gene. In rodents, lack of leptin increases appetite, but in humans deficiency of it is rare – so giving extra leptin to obese people rarely works. Indeed, they normally have high leptin levels, as they have more adipose tissue, and the hormone is stored in body fat. It may be, however, that obese people are resistant to leptin (as many are to insulin) and this may affect appetite, resulting in weight gain.

Meanwhile, there's interesting research on the body chemical dopamine, which, with the other neurotransmitters, including serotonin and norepinephrine (noradrenaline), helps regulate appetite and is linked with our pleasure in food. Available dopamine seems to be reduced in obese people who eat compulsively. There may soon be drugs based on leptin and/or dopamine to help beat overeating. Meanwhile, scientists have found exercise helps increase the body's sensitivity to both.

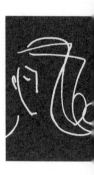

Eating slowly can help moderate appetite, as the brain takes about 10 minutes to register feelings of fullness. Fatty, sugary foods are worst, as they're eaten quicker. Eating more frequently can also help control appetite by regulating blood sugar, and it's best if small frequent meals contain low GI foods (see Question 66). Appetite may also be blunted by drinking a large glass of water.

Appetite can also be controlled by some prescription drugs (see Question 34) and herbal diet supplements.

Q21

Why is weight easier to gain than lose?

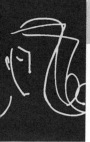

When you reduce calorie intake, as a protection against starvation the body reduces its metabolic rate. (There may also be a 'set point' factor, see Question 10.) The reduction also makes sense as, after losing weight for a while, you will naturally have a lower BMR (Question 5). After crash dieting, the body loses a proportionately high amount of lean tissue, which can also reduce metabolic rate.

On a negative-energy diet (fewer calories eaten than expended), the normal pattern is first to lose weight at the expected rate (1lb/450g for every 3,500 calories' deficit). Soon, though, weight loss slows because the metabolic rate is slowing. The answer is to increase energy expenditure and lean muscle mass as discussed, and perhaps reduce calorie intake further.

It sometimes seems pounds come on overnight, but if you suddenly eat a lot after slimming, the body retains more fluid and it's this, not fat, that's gained. Even a total blowout is unlikely to put on more than a pound of fat. Psychology plays a part – as long as you feel 'eating is nice' and 'dieting is bad', you'll find it hard to lose weight.

you and your body

Q22

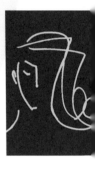

A study of American female nurses showed overall mortality increased in an almost exact line with weight. Research at St Thomas's Hospital in 2005 found that being overweight – especially when under 30 – adds almost 9 years to a woman's biological age, by accelerating cell damage from free radicals.

However, if you are a stone heavier than you'd like but are healthy, fit and well, and your BMI (see Question 26) is within healthy limits, then it may be best simply to ensure you don't put on too much more. Especially try to keep from developing an 'apple' shape, as central fat distribution is an indicator of increased risk of several conditions.

A reasonable covering of body fat has advantages – it's insulating and protective, it secretes the hormone leptin, which boosts the immune system, it may help mood, and is essential for puberty and reproduction, and important in menopausal and older women. That's not to say overweight is necessary for these functions, or that it should be taken lightly. Gross overweight coupled with a lack of regular activity is a recipe for disaster.

you and your body

As you get older is
weight gain natural
or even desirable?

The UK National Sizing Survey found people put on weight
from 25 until their mid-to-late 50s and then typically start to
shrink. The heaviest women were aged 45 to 54, while
men's weight peaked at 55 to 64. The main reason for this
gain is that as we age our muscle mass declines through
inactivity and the ageing process. Between the ages of 30
and 70, muscle strength and mass decrease by about 30%.

Our metabolic rate – the rate at which we burn calories
– is largely dependent upon our proportion of lean tissue
(muscle) and with its loss the result is slowing of the
metabolism. Hormonal changes – e.g. to thyroid and
adrenal function, etc. – can also slow it. To counteract this,
and maintain a steady weight, calorie intake would need to
be gradually reduced. (As a rough guide, around 100
calories a day for every decade over 30. So, if you're, say,
60 you need 300 calories fewer than at 30, if you don't
exercise). This generally doesn't happen and the result is a
positive energy balance – extra fat stores on the body!

In theory, however, this process can be blunted.
Research shows that, with regular activity and weight

training, lean tissue loss can be reduced by about half and cardiovascular function largely maintained, which also helps maintain optimum metabolic rate. Hormonal changes may also be minimized with regular exercise.

Research on élite runners aged 50 to 70 (about the fittest people for their age) shows that however hard you work, body composition and shape will change with age – albeit much more slowly. The athletes' lean tissue decreased by an average of about $5\frac{1}{2}$ lb (half normal average), body fat percentage increased by 5% and waist size by about 2 inches, but they didn't put on weight.

This probably means that, for most of us taking reasonable exercise, we should regard moderate changes in shape and small weight increases as natural as we age – the amount dependent upon how much exercise we do and how well we balance calorie intake with expenditure. Huge weight increases are not natural and are connected more with social and environmental factors.

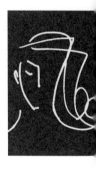

A reasonably small weight gain may well be desirable if you were thin when younger – for example, thin people are more prone to osteoporosis in later life. Body fat stores may help to keep oestrogen levels up, which in turn helps protect bones. As a guide, from 50 into old age, a BMI at the high end of desirable may be wiser. So, as we age a small weight gain is natural and may be good in some respects, whereas large gains – or losses – are neither natural nor good and are linked with increased risk of heart disease. Several studies have linked low calorie intake – especially in midlife – with much reduced risk of heart disease and a longer lifespan.

Q24

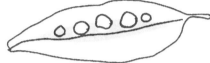

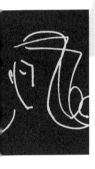

The basic classification is Body Mass Index (see Question 26), which is used worldwide, but interpreted differently. The World Health Organization describes normal weight as a BMI of 18.5–24.99, overweight 25+; BMIs of 18–25 are associated with lowest risk of death. Others say a BMI of up to 27 is acceptable, as health risks don't really show until then. However, these figures are not 100% reliable, as they take no account of body composition. For example, an athlete with high muscle mass and low body fat might have a BMI over 25. There is also obviously room for large differences in weight between people of the same height. Perhaps halfway between 20 and 25 could be considered 'perfect' – a BMI of 22.5 – an idea endorsed by the American Heart Association. Others feel such guidelines are too specific. There's really no such thing as a perfect weight for everyone at every time in their lives.

Another gauge of weight is body-fat percentage (see Question 27). Waist size should also be considered, as a disproportionately large midriff is an indicator of increased health risks.

you and your body

42

**Is there any very
quick and easy way
to tell if I'm
overweight?**

The 10-second test: you get a very good indication of
whether you're health-risk-related overweight by
measuring your waist. If over 34.5in (88cm) for females
or 40in (102cm) for males, then you're almost certainly
overweight.

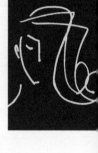

You can also try the 'pinch test' – if you can pinch a
fold of flesh around your midriff at least 1 inch (2.5cm)
thick, you're probably overweight (not exactly
scientific).

Another quick rule-of-thumb is, if you were at an ideal
weight (BMI 22–23) at age 25, add 5lb (2.25kg) for every
decade and you can assume you're not overweight. For
example, at 55 you could be 15lb (6.75kg) heavier than
at 25, and consider your weight as within acceptable
bounds.

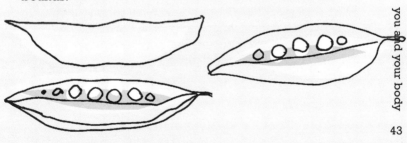

you and your body

What exactly is Body Mass Index (BMI) and how do I calculate it?

The Body Mass Index is a formula used by health professionals worldwide to assess body weight in relation to height. It's a useful measure, because in most people it correlates with body-fat percentage. However, some sportspeople, pregnant or lactating women, very elderly or frail people shouldn't use it, and it shouldn't be used for children (see Question 275).

BMI = weight in kilograms divided by height in metres (squared). To get your weight in kilograms, divide weight in pounds by 2.2. To get your height in metres, multiply height in inches by 0.025. Squared height is height multiplied by itself (e.g. 1.65 x 1.65 = 2.72).

BMI UNDER 18.5: UNDERWEIGHT – You don't need to lose weight and, although your risk of having health problems associated with obesity is very low, you may be at increased risk of other problems such as bone loss, nutrient deficiency and others.

BMI 18.5–24.99: NORMAL – You don't need to lose or gain weight. You're within healthy guidelines and risk of weight-related health problems is minimal. The 'ideal'

you and your body

44

BMI is between 22 and 23 for young adults. At the upper range of normal (around 24.99), if you feel you're overweight, do the waist test (Question 25) as an additional check. If at the upper end and have been gaining weight steadily at more than 5lb (2.25kg) per decade over age 25, you might pay more attention to diet and exercise levels and aim to put no more on, or at least slow rate of increase.

BMI 25–29.99: OVERWEIGHT (PRE-OBESE) – From a BMI of 25 up to around 27, you have a slightly increased risk of health problems (some experts call this the 'caution zone'). Using the waist test (Question 25) will give a clearer idea whether you have cause for concern. Ensure your weight doesn't increase further. From over 27, risk of health problems becomes higher. In one study, a measurable increased incidence of high blood pressure, heart disease and diabetes was noted at 27.3 for women and 27.8 for men. For many within this category it would be advisable to get BMI down to at least 25–27.

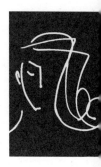

BMI 30–34.99: OBESE CLASS 1 – You're officially 'obese' (very overweight) and your risk of weight-related diseases increases considerably, especially if you have a large waist (see Question 25). Reducing weight by even 5% or 10% would give considerable health benefits.

BMI 35–40: OBESE CLASS 2 – Risk of death and weight-related health problems increases considerably, defined as 'severe'. It's important to reduce BMI.

BMI OVER 40: OBESE CLASS 3 (EXTREME OR MORBID OBESITY) – An extremely high risk of early death and weight-related health problems. It is very important to reduce BMI; your doctor can refer you for specialist help.

Q27

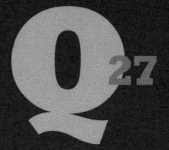

What is 'body-fat percentage' and how does it relate to my weight?

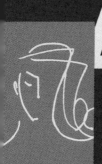

Body-fat percentage is the proportion of adipose (fat) tissue in your body by weight. Question 1 has more detail. When you gain weight, the increase is nearly all due to increase in adipose fat; i.e., body-fat percentage gets higher while lean tissue (muscle) remains fairly static.

For adult men, average body-fat percentage is 15–20%, (overweight would be over about 25% and obesity over about 30%), while for adult women average is about 25–27% (overweight over about 30% and obesity over about 35%). In very overweight people, body-fat percentage can rise as high as 70%. In very fit people, body-fat percentages of around 10% for males and 20% for females are more normal.

It isn't possible to measure body-fat percentage very accurately without professional equipment. However, you can buy scales that include a body-fat calculator, or professional body-fat monitors. For the average person, it is not vital to work out body-fat percentage, as BMI (Question 26) and waist measurement (Question 25) will do a satisfactory job of deciding if you're overweight.

Q28

Can dieting slow my metabolic rate?

If you lose weight, your metabolic rate decreases, mostly because your body has less to do (carrying less weight) and so uses fewer calories. Other factors being equal, you need to eat less to maintain that weight. (If you put weight back on, your metabolic rate rises again.)

Other factors may be involved. As in Question 21, the body seems to defend high weight more than low, so a 3,500-calorie intake reduction doesn't always translate to 1lb fat loss. So weight loss will become progressively harder as metabolic rate slows more than might be predicted.

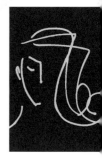

People taking regular physical activity, including aerobic and strength training, find dieting doesn't alter the metabolism so much. Regular aerobic exercise can raise metabolic rate for hours afterwards. Weight training will also help dieters avoid lean tissue loss and may even add some. Being heavier and using more calories than fat, a good proportion of lean tissue is essential to good metabolic rate. Crash or very-low-cal diets tend to lose a high proportion of it; whereas moderate energy restriction loses proportionately more fat, so steady slimming is best.

you and your body

47

Q29

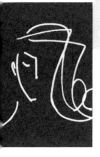

If long-term calorie reduction made people fat, then people in famines would be fat. It is obvious that if you don't get enough to eat, you will lose weight, not gain it.

If you create a long-term energy deficit, expending more energy than you ingest in the form of calories, then you will definitely lose weight. It's always best if conscious 'dieting' is combined with regular exercise of various types and if the dieting is done in a steady manner.

There is evidence to show that repeated bouts of 'yo-yo' dieting may make it ever harder to lose weight, but this is probably to do with the fact that repeated dieting tends to deplete lean tissue (muscle) and each time weight is regained the lost lean tissue isn't replaced unless muscle-building exercise is done. Over time this would mean that the metabolic rate would be reduced, as lean tissue is more metabolically active than fat. Severe crash dieting may also deplete more lean tissue than slow dieting.

The answer is to avoid yo-yo and crash dieting and to get plenty of muscle-enhancing exercise, whether slimming or attempting to maintain your weight.

you and your body

48

Q30

Will my percentage of body fat increase each time I diet?

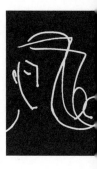

When you diet to lose weight you should decrease your percentage of body fat. However, the question implies that you're a yo-yo (sometimes called 'weight cycling') dieter and it is probably true that, with repeated bouts of yo-yoing, every time you return to a high weight, your percentage of total fat may have increased a little.

This is because, when you lose weight, some of the weight loss is lean tissue (particularly if you crash diet) and, when you put weight back on, lean tissue isn't replaced. So you'll be your old weight, but have less lean tissue and thus may have a slightly higher percentage of body fat. Compared with the last time you were at this same high weight, your overall resting metabolism will have decreased slightly because of the lower proportion of lean tissue (see previous question). So this time it may be a little harder to lose weight.

Avoid yo-yo and crash dieting, and always exercise when slimming to retain as much lean tissue (muscle) as you can.

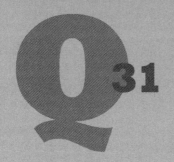

**Can I lose weight
without dieting?**

You can create a small long-term calorie deficit or
negative energy balance by increasing the amount of
exercise you do to 'burn up' calories, and this will be
enough alone to help you lose weight slowly over time,
all other factors being equal (e.g. as long as you don't
begin to eat more). In one study, a group of people who
didn't diet but increased exercise levels lost about 6lb
(2.75kg) over a year.

The amount you could lose like this would be about
1lb (0.5kg) for every 3,500 calories you burn up over
and above your current rate. To burn an extra 3,500
calories over a week, i.e. 500 a day, would be possible.
However, even an extra 200 calories burnt every day
would produce weight loss over time.

The only other ways to lose body fat without 'dieting'
(i.e. reducing your calorie intake to create a negative
energy balance) are to have surgery such as liposuction
or to take pills to speed up the metabolic rate. Some
prescription slimming pills will do this, but others still
require you to eat less and help by reducing appetite.

you and your body

50

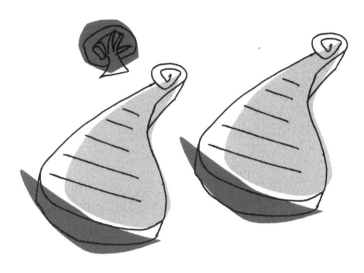

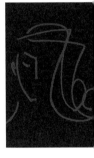

Questions 33 and 34 discuss these options further. You can lose weight that is body fluid by taking diuretics, but these should only be taken under medical advice, and it is pointless if you are trying to lose fat.

However, if by 'dieting' you mean 'following a set or crash diet', then it is perfectly possible to lose weight by altering eating patterns, rather than 'going on a diet'. Several studies have shown that a healthy low-fat, high-carbohydrate diet of around 1,500 calories a day (much higher than in many diets) produces the best long-term weight loss, and that crash dieting is, indeed, a waste of time. So, if you don't like the word diet, don't use it.

Q32

What's the best way to lose weight?

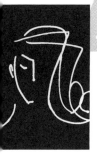

By both reducing your calorie intake a little (for most people around 500 calories fewer a day is a good average to aim for) and increasing your regular activity.

There's probably no such thing as an absolute best for the way either to reduce calories or to exercise – both vary according to your tastes, weight, means, health, etc. The answers for you personally should become more apparent if you read through this book, which aims to look at all the options.

In general terms, though, it seems that the most successful long-term weight-loss programmes involve reduction in total fat and simple carbohydrate intake, thus reducing total calorie intake, as well as eating (at a slow speed) regular meals containing plenty of fruit and vegetables. It also seems the most popular and easy way to increase energy output is regular walking.

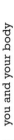

you and your body

52

Q33

Are there any operations I can have to make me lose weight?

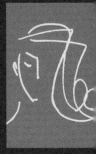

Perhaps the best-known operation now is liposuction – a process that 'sucks' the fat from your body through a tube. It is the only operation, as far as I know, that actually removes your body fat – but it is usually not such a 'minor' operation as some people would have you believe.

Other operations rely upon reducing the amount that you can eat, or by preventing the absorption of foods, or a combination of the two. All of these operations are available privately, but may also be available in the UK via the NHS if you are a suitable case. However, they are not to be undertaken as anything except a last resort for the obese, as they have life-changing consequences, not all positive.

One other type of operation is an abdominoplasty, which is really for the post-obese person who has a lot of loose 'spare' skin hanging around. The operation cuts away the loose flesh. See your GP for a discussion about your options regarding surgery.

Is it a good idea to take slimming pills?

The World Health Organization describes prescription slimming pills as 'an adjunct to other weight-loss therapies and a way of helping to maintain body weight over time'. It does also point out that these drugs are best used in conjunction with diet and lifestyle management, and that when such drugs are discontinued weight regain occurs.

It goes without saying that prescription slimming pills should be used under medical supervision. Current UK criteria are that intervention with drugs should only be applied after a minimum 3 months' 'lifestyle intervention' and a weight loss of 10% already achieved. However, these guidelines aren't always followed. Normally you shouldn't be given prescription slimming drugs unless you have a BMI of at least 30 or weight-related health problems.

Two drugs are most likely to be prescribed. One is orlistat (brand name Xenical), which works by blocking absorption of about one-third of the fat in food. Patients are required to follow a low-fat diet anyway (otherwise complications like 'leaky bowel' may occur). Guidelines for prescribing orlistat in the UK are that you should be 18

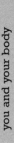

you and your body

to 75, have lost 2.5kg (5½lb) in the previous month and have a BMI of at least 28. The other drug is sibutramine (Reductil in the UK and Meridia in the USA), which acts by both inhibiting appetite and stimulating metabolic rate. Possible side effects include raised blood pressure, and, as it is fairly new, long-term effects are uncertain.

An exciting new drug, rimonabant (brand name Acomplia), which works by helping regulate food intake, is due to become available on prescription in mid 2006. Acomplia is especially good at reducing central body fat. Phentermine is another drug that stimulates the central nervous system and is used as an appetite suppressant.

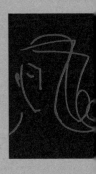

Are slimming drugs a good idea? I wouldn't presume to judge, but certainly the message seems to be that they are only to be considered for a small proportion of overweight people. The decision of whether you are a suitable patient is best left to a doctor or specialist who knows you. So I wouldn't recommend you visit a private doctor who has never met you before; private slimming clinics across the world offer pills at a price – which could include your health.

However, scientists worldwide are working hard to find a slimming pill that is safe and effective – recently there have been reported an injection that kills fat cells, a gene which stops mice making fat cells, and the uncoupling protein 'UPC-3', which can turn surplus calories directly into heat rather than fat. A variety of non-prescription slimming pills with varying degrees of usefulness are sold, the best of which is probably Zotrim, a combination of South American herbs.

Q35 Why do so many people put weight back on after they've dieted?

All the research agrees with you – that the majority of slimmers do regain their lost weight. About 10% of slimmers will have retained their new slim weight after 9 months, only about 5% after several years. Some research (but not all) says that after 5 years almost everyone returns to or goes higher than their starting weight. Sadly, new research by the British Dietetic Association finds that in the long run a third of dieters end up anything up to a stone heavier.

The main reason is usually that calorie intake gradually creeps up and because, as we've seen (in Questions 3, 21, 28, 29 and 30), a slim person has a slower metabolic rate than a fat person, calorie intake needs to be restricted permanently if the new weight is to remain. This should not mean that a newly slim person should have to remain on a 'slimming-level' diet for life, but certainly that a calorie intake lower than pre-diet levels is needed. Many people find it hard to continue with this more restrained way of eating.

The best way to keep weight off permanently is to take more exercise, but again many slimmers are reluctant to do this. In other words, ex-slimmers find that their lifestyle just isn't conducive to the permanent changes necessary for permanent weight loss. However, there is some brighter news. A very recent American study of ex-WeightWatchers slimmers found that 5 years later over 70% were still below their original weight and nearly 20% were within 5lb (2kg) of their original goal weight. Again in America, the National Weight Control Registry recruited 784 people who had maintained at least a 30lb (13.5kg) weight loss for an average of $5\frac{1}{2}$ years. Most had a genetic background (e.g. fat parents) that might be assumed to predispose them to overweight, and, indeed, many had been overweight since childhood, but still managed to keep the weight off.

**How can I avoid
regaining all the
weight I've lost?**

First of all, let's hope that you've settled on a reasonable
'target' weight, which is always easier to maintain than
one that's too low. For young adults, a target BMI of
around 22 to 23 is as low as you want to go – but 25
would be fine if your starting level was higher than 28,
especially if you are over 40. For older adults, a target
BMI of around 24–25 is often reasonable. Use your
common sense. If you go too low, you will need to reduce
your regular calorie intake down low as well, and this
may be too hard to do (see the previous question).

Secondly, let's hope that you dieted slowly so that you
didn't lose too much lean tissue (muscle). The more
muscle you have on your body, the more calories you will
burn up every day rather than storing them as fat.
Research shows that very fast (crash) dieting does lose
more lean tissue than slow dieting.

Thirdly, you need to eat a healthy balanced diet and
keep the total fat content fairly low, while filling your
plate with more of the complex carbohydrates,
vegetables, fruits and low-fat proteins. You need to eat

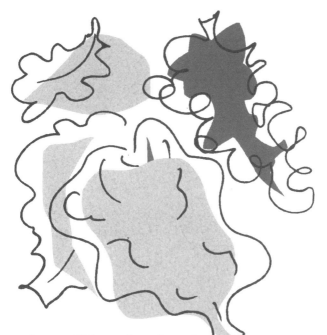

regular smallish meals and snacks – portion control is a simple method of watching total calorie intake.

Fourthly, look at your lifestyle and try to adjust it so that you are less inclined to overeat (see pages 154–237).

Last, but definitely not least, you need to take regular exercise – preferably both aerobic (e.g. walking, cycling) and weight training (e.g. with free weights or at a gym). The people mentioned in the last paragraph of the previous question, who kept their weight off for at least 5 years, almost all cited regular exercise, such as brisk walking, or dancing, sport or gym work, as the main reason.

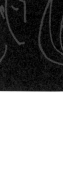

Q37 What factors affect my body shape?

Your shape is largely governed by your parents' genes – you take bits from both parents to make up your own unique self – but exactly how you will end up is, of course, a bit of a lottery! For example, if you have a father who is tall and thin and a mother who is short and plump, your genetic shape could be short and thin, or tall and plump, as well as tall and thin or short and plump. You could even end up neither short nor tall, and neither thin nor plump, because if you put short and tall together you get medium, and so on.

If you're lucky, you could take all the 'best bits' from each parent and end up completely gorgeous, even though neither of them is particularly handsome. That's why siblings can look so different – apart from identical twins, you each put your parents' genes into a different pattern. As you probably know, however, children from the same family usually do have many physical similarities and bear strong characteristics from one or other parent.

Other factors do come into the equation, though.

Obviously, your gender has a large bearing upon your shape, because each sex is genetically programmed to have a predisposition to its own blueprint of muscle, bone, fat and so on. Males tend to have broader shoulders, wider necks, narrower hips and more muscled arms and legs – and tend to be taller with a lower percentage of body fat. Females tend to have higher body fat, deposited around the breasts, hips, bottom and thighs – with a lower percentage of muscle and tending to be shorter. Male and female hormones decide these sexual differences but, again, everyone has both male and female hormones in them and, depending upon the proportion of each that you have, your shape can be more or less mannish or more or less feminine.

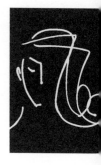

Your shape can also be affected by your nutritional status in early life (see the last question) and also, to quite a reasonable extent, by what and how much activity you do and have done. For example, look how different are the figures of a body builder, a gymnast, a marathon runner and a rugby player. Exercise has a quite tremendous power to help shape your body. Though, of course, people tend to choose the sport that fits in best with their original body blueprint – i.e. if you are tall, broad and powerful you are more likely to become a rugby player than a gymnast.

Weight is less of a factor in defining body shape than you may think, though being fat will accentuate shape. For example, a fat pear-shaped woman looks more pear-shaped than a thin pear-shaped woman.

Q38

I am female, with bulky arm and leg muscles – even though I do hardly any exercise. How can I get rid of them?

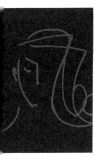

You sound like a classic mesomorph (see Question 40), and you are going to find it nearly impossible to turn yourself into a thin ectomorph or a rounded endomorph. However, some people with these body types would probably give a lot to be more like you. You can probably eat more or less what you want without getting fat and you are, no doubt, strong and fit as well, with good bone mass – all positives. What you may be able to do is streamline yourself with stretching exercises and/or yoga.

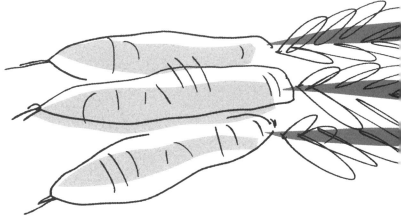

you and your body

62

Q39

What about spot-reduction – can I choose where I lose fat via exercise?

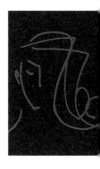

It's been said you can lose fat in specific places by working the muscles over them (the idea being that the muscle burns extra fat there). However, research shows this isn't the case. A study measuring subcutaneous fat in tennis players' arms found the fat underneath the (more muscular) playing arm was exactly the same as under the other arm. Body fat can only be reduced by creating an energy deficit (see Question 15) and using stored fat this way – you can't dictate from where you want fat to go.

Research shows fat tends to go first from the face, bust and abdomen – and, indeed, the intra-abdominal adipose tissue is easier to mobilize than that elsewhere in the body, particularly the hips and thighs. Hence, if you have a fat middle, it may appear you're spot-reducing, as this area will show the most marked changes initially.

Toning exercises can improve your appearance in specific areas by streamlining or flattening the area where the muscle is worked, giving you a better shape. This achieves a similar effect to spot-reducing and may be where the original misconception came from.

you and your body

Q40

How can I best work with my particular body shape?

Broadly speaking, bodies can be categorized into one of three basic shapes. Some people are very true to type, but most of us may be near to one type but take some characteristics from another. Whichever you are nearest to, it is best to work 'with' it rather than 'against' it.

ECTOMORPH: The ectomorph body is tall and thin, looks 'narrow' and, usually, delicate. This type of person will probably find it hard to put on weight because of a high metabolic rate. Muscle profile may be low or moderate and can be improved with weight training. Body fat content will be lower than average and contours are sharp and angular. The ectomorph is suited to long-distance running, basketball and a variety of other sports in which limb length and light weight are advantages. In later life, an ectomorph may be predisposed to putting on weight around the abdomen.

MESOMORPH: The mesomorph is well built, with well-muscled arms and legs and a general appearance of power. Male mesomorphs are the closest body type to the

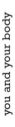

classic 'V' shape, with powerful shoulders and chest, and slim midriff. Mesomorphs have a higher muscle-to-body-fat ratio than most and will be suited to sprinting, football, gymnastics and many other activities. Mesomorphs can eat plenty, as they usually like to keep active and their high proportion of lean tissue means their metabolic rate will be high. In later life they may do less and put on body fat.

ENDOMORPH: The endomorph body is rounded, with a soft appearance. There is a higher-than-average body-fat percentage and muscle mass may be proportionately low. They may find that excess body fat accumulates easily and this may be compounded by a lack of interest in, or aptitude for, physical exercise. The endomorph will never be an ectomorph, but it is possible – with determination – to put on lean tissue, maintain weight at a healthy level and enjoy several forms of activity, such as walking or swimming. The endomorph should take care to avoid putting on too much weight, especially in midlife.

Aren't endomorphs just fat ectomorphs or out-of-condition mesomorphs? No, it's not as simple as that. If you were to visit a maternity unit, you would quickly see that when babies are born they really do all have their own shapes and sizes, even within the same family. Have a look at photos of yourself soon after birth and you should be able to spot your basic type from that. Sure, some mesomorphs can adopt endo-characteristics and some ectos may, in time, put on weight, but your basic type is what you were born with and what, mostly, you will stay with.

Q41 I've slimmed down to a weight I love, but I hate my flat and shapeless bum. Any ideas?

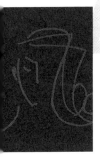

You can improve a flat bum through both posture – standing correctly will immediately tighten and raise the bum (see Question 43) – and regular 'gluteal' exercise, which will improve the size and shape of the buttocks a lot. Parallel squats and leg lifts will help. A low-cost step platform is a good home investment for the glutes (as long as you use it!). At the gym, the step machine, the exercise bikes and the seated leg press will help. Stepping exercise classes are good. Outdoors, uphill walking, skiing and cycling are beneficial. Other sports that give you a good bum are dancing, ice skating and gymnastics. To see improvement, you need to do whatever combination of these that you choose regularly.

I've also heard of bottom implants from the US – like breast implants but larger. Before you consider this, however, remember that for many women a small bottom is the Holy Grail... and clothes do hang better if you have a slim behind!

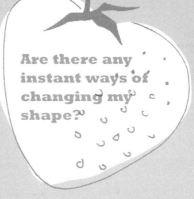

Are there any instant ways of changing my shape?

The best 'instant' way is by standing correctly (see Question 43) – poor posture has a lot to answer for in terms of round shoulders, double chins, fat bellies, flat bottoms and knock-knees (for example)! I suppose you could change some facets of your shape (e.g. fat stomach, big thighs) through liposuction – sometimes a painful process. It's not exactly instant but it does involve little effort on your part (apart from the work involved in earning the money to pay for it). For a special occasion, you could also try a salon wrap for a quick but short-lived minor change in your body measurements and there are now several hold-in type garments, including pants, tights and swimwear that claim to help you look up to a stone thinner instantly.

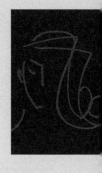

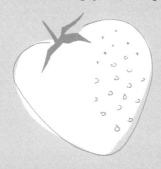

you and your body

How can posture help?

You can actually make bits of your body look better – even disappear – by simply standing or sitting correctly! Look half a stone lighter just by adjusting your body alignment. This could be the only 'instant miracle' in this book.

Poor posture can contribute to several problems, such as double chin, fat belly or 'dropped' bottom. Mostly, poor posture comes over time, encouraged by poor lifestyle habits – slouching, hunching over desks, taking too little exercise, etc. Poor body alignment is also associated with headaches, neck pain, backache, and general aches, as well as tiredness/lack of energy. Good posture isn't only important for shape, it can help you feel better.

Over years of misuse, muscles governing posture can become too short, stiff and tight, or too long and weak – so if you find correct posture difficult, you need exercises to help them back into shape. This may take some weeks...!

CORRECTING POSTURE:
• With the upper body held correctly – shoulders relaxed and down, chest wide, neck balanced on spine so the ears

line up with the shoulders – a double chin is minimized.
• When shoulders and spine are held correctly, the
bustline becomes higher.
• When pelvis and spine are in perfect alignment and the
bottom tucked in, a 'pot belly' can virtually disappear –
but it takes toned abdominal muscles to maintain this
position for longer than a minute or so.
• The basis of good posture is the correct tilt of the pelvis.
If tipped too far forward, the stomach sticks out, the lower
back has too great a curve and the spine is thrown out of
alignment. If the pelvis is tipped too far back, the lower
spine will be too rigid and flat. If aligned correctly, good
posture follows naturally. Stand at a mirror and practise
tilting your pelvis into the correct position, keeping the
knees slightly relaxed – you'll feel your ribcage naturally
'opening' as you do so. Maintain this even while sitting.
• Strong abdominals and correct pelvic tilt lift and 'tighten'
the bottom by making the gluteal muscles work. This also
helps correct knock-knees and flat feet.
• With correct posture you may be up to an inch taller.
• Remember your posture as you stand chatting on the
phone, stand in a queue, etc. These hours really add up
and can make a huge difference.
• Also sit properly – at work, in front of the TV, etc. Check
regularly that your spine and pelvis are in neutral and
your head well balanced on your spine, with no muscle
tension in the neck and shoulders.
• Yoga, Pilates and the Alexander Technique can all help
you to gain better posture, as can many exercise classes,
such as stretch and body conditioning.

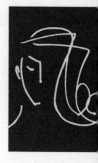

you and your body

Q44

Is it true that a pear shape is the hardest shape of all to change?

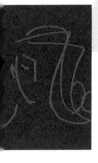

This is a typically female shape, as oestrogen hormones present in highest quantities in females predispose to fat stores in the hips, thighs and bottom. This seems to be the hardest of all body fat to 'mobilize' when an energy deficit is created (fewer calories in than expended) and this probably evolved so females had good fat stores for pregnancy and breastfeeding. In both men and women, studies have concluded that fat comes off the body from the top downwards, so to a 'pear' it can seem as if the fat never moves off the hips and thighs.

Hence, the pear shape IS hardest to change. Not all women are 'pears'– indeed, some men are – but if you are, you're basically stuck with it. Even if you manage to lose weight, you will still be a slimmed-down pear shape, as your top half will have slimmed too. No diet or exercise plan will get rid of fat just off your lower body. However, exercise can tone up large hips, thighs and bottom and this can improve pear appearance. Some resort to liposuction, which has its drawbacks.

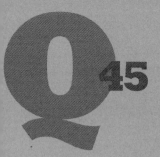

Q45

**Can I spot-reduce
my hips and thighs
by dieting?**

No. When you create an energy deficit, by eating less
and/or increasing exercise output, in general terms you
will lose weight from all over. People who follow 'hip
and thigh'-type diets also lose inches from their waist,
bust and so on. In fact a 'hip and thigh'-type diet will
probably seem to have more of an effect on the stomach
at first, because body fat apparently shifts first from the
face, bust (or chest) and stomach, and last from the hips
and thighs (see the previous question). People wanting
to spot-reduce their stomachs will appear to have more
success because of this – and research does show that
abdominal fat is easier to shift. It's not fair for the pear-
shaped person, but see Question 46 if you want to be
cheered up.

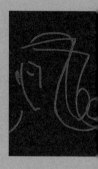

Q46

Is it true that if overweight is mostly on the lower half of the body it is perfectly healthy?

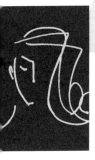

Nearly right. Very many research studies show that surplus weight concentrated around the abdomen (intra-abdominal fat, central fat distribution) is much more of a health risk than evenly distributed general overweight; also that heavy hips and thighs in women are normal, not a weight 'problem' (see Question 44). It is because of this that some health professionals are now beginning to pay more attention to the waist test (see Question 25) when judging overweight than to the Body Mass Index (see Question 26).

So, if you have a lot of weight on your hips and thighs but an average waist circumference – even if your BMI says that you are overweight – then you're probably not overweight at all! It is only if your waist is 'at risk' too, and/or your BMI is much over the normal range, that you may indeed be an overweight and at-risk pear.

Q47

What is an apple shape and why is it unhealthy?

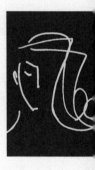

An apple-shaped person tends to store fat around the abdomen, chest and upper arms, giving the shape of an apple. It has been found that this has a higher link with several health problems, including diabetes and CHD (coronary heart disease), than other shapes (e.g. pear) because 'central' body fat produces chemicals, proteins and hormones that may damage the insulin system, raise blood pressure and increase blood cholesterol.

Indeed, even if the scales – or your BMI (see Question 26) – don't say you're overweight, but you have sufficient apple shape to give a waist measurement over 37in (94cm) for men or $31^{1}/_{2}$in (80cm) for women, then you have an increased health risk. The National Obesity Forum says waist measurement can predict the risk of Type 2 diabetes and heart disease more accurately than weight.

So, if you're an apple, it's important to make lifestyle changes to get your middle under control. As a bonus, you will also look a nicer shape. The good news is that intra-abdominal fat seems to be more cooperative in disappearing than lower-body fat.

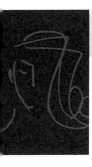

If you diet to lose weight, you will lose a little fat off your legs (and arms, and indeed elsewhere), but if you are the classic apple shape, with a round fat stomach and thin arms and legs, the fat loss on your limbs will hardly show compared with the amount of difference you'll notice on your middle. Apples are lucky in this way because the abdominal fat is usually not that hard to shift.

You should also combine the diet with exercise to trim your abdomen and add muscle – and therefore shape – to your limbs. If you're out of condition, do this first and then you could move on to a weight-training programme. Regular aerobic work, like cycling and/or rowing, will also help. At the end of all this, you should look more in proportion.

Q49

What's the best way to get a firm, flat stomach?

Lose weight if necessary – muscles won't show through fat – and do lots of regular abdominal work, exercising not only the 'six pack' muscle running the length of your abdomen, but also the obliques to either side and 'core' muscles that lie across the region.

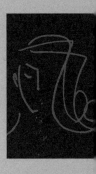

You only need a few different exercises to work all these areas, but do them slowly and well. If stomach floor exercises hurt your neck, use an abdominal cage, which can be inexpensive. Yoga and Pilates will also help.

Your stomach is often the first area to slacken, as it doesn't get exercised much in the course of sedentary life. To target abs during your normal day, try getting up from chairs without using your hands, walk uphill and downhill (or stairs) when you can, and do this exercise (you may not want to if you have high blood pressure):

Sit in the correct pelvic tilt position (see Question 43); draw in your abdomen, concentrating on the area below your navel. Pull in as hard as you can, breathing normally, and hold for a count of 5. Relax and repeat whenever you remember.

My bust is too big – can I reduce it through diet and exercise, without losing weight from the rest of my body?

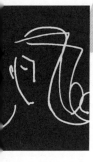

As you'll see if you read the answers to Questions 39, 45 and 48, the idea of spot-reducing or gaining fat on any one particular part of the body is a bit of a myth, with the exception that when you lose weight over time, it tends first to come off the face, bust and stomach. So I suppose if you lose a small amount of weight there is a chance that your bust will get smaller (along with your face and stomach) and, if you then stop at that point, the rest of your body will stay the same. However, this isn't an exact science. No exercise can reduce your bust, I'm afraid. If it is really very large and is causing you problems, I suggest you see your doctor and ask him to refer you to a specialist for further advice.

Q51

My face is fat and yet I'm quite slim – is there anything I can do about this?

I am afraid if your face is naturally round and full, even though you aren't overweight, you can't diet your face thin, and there aren't any facial exercises you could do to remove fat either (see the questions about spot-reducing: 39, 45 and 50). I have heard of people having liposuction on their face and even removing teeth to give themselves hollow cheeks, but this seems somewhat drastic. If you really don't like your cheeks, your make-up (if you happen to be female) and hairstyle can go a long way to disguising this. I'm also told that as you age the face is likely to thin down.

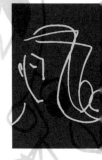

Q52

I have a month to get in shape before my holiday – what can I hope to achieve?

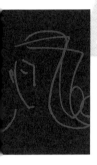

If you need to lose a little weight, you could probably lose about half a stone (3kg) without resorting to a crash-type diet. If you need to lose a lot more, you could probably lose a few pounds more. If you do regular weight-training and aerobic exercise (say, every other day), you could firm your stomach, slim down your waist a little, and improve posture and the appearance of your arms, legs and bottom.

How much is really up to you, your own body, how hard you work and so on. If you're really out of condition, however, you definitely shouldn't go 'mad' to try to get in shape – you could injure muscles or tendons, strain your back, you may feel exhausted, have headaches, and so on. Even if you only do very mild toning work, if you start today and do it regularly – at least 3 times a week – you'll definitely look and feel a bit better by your holiday. Don't forget to continue your programme during the holiday and when it is over.

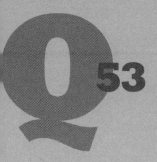

Q 53

Do you recommend a salon wrap or similar treatment to help lose weight in a hurry?

What you will get from most salon wraps is temporary inch loss from the wrapped areas. You will no doubt be measured at several strategic points before you are 'wrapped' and again afterwards, and the salon will add up the small losses and tell you that you have lost x number of inches altogether. This will probably sound more impressive than it actually is. However, you will probably find that the abdomen and waist area reduce the most, and this might be useful if you wanted to wear a special, slightly tight dress, for instance. Normally, after an evening of eating and drinking, most of the benefit of the wrap will disappear. It's only a temporary solution, as what has 'disappeared' is fluid not fat. No wrap can get rid of your fat for you; you need to create an energy deficit to do that.

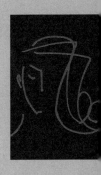

Q54

Now I'm slimmer, how can I exercise away skin left from when I was very fat?

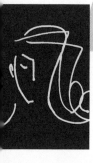

If you have lost a great deal of weight, these skin folds can be very hard, if not impossible, to shift, especially if you were overweight for a long time and/or are older. It might be a good idea to see your doctor, as it is possible to remove the surplus skin via an operation called an abdominoplasty. You would be a good candidate as you are now down to target weight. You can also have such an operation done privately.

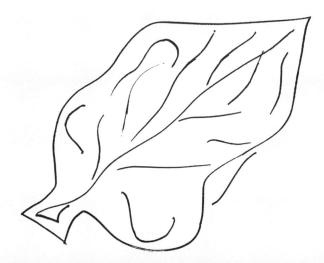

Q55

What is the best exercise for making myself look taller and slimmer?

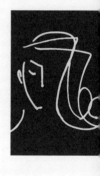

Good posture is the best starting point – see Question 43. Then any exercise that involves stretching will help you to look taller, as your muscles are streamlined. Examples are a stretching routine or class, yoga, Pilates and the Alexander Technique. Toning exercises will help you to look slimmer by flattening out the areas that most people don't like – a tummy bulge is a perfect example.

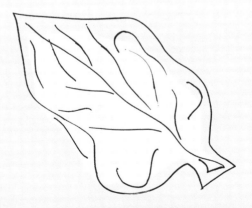

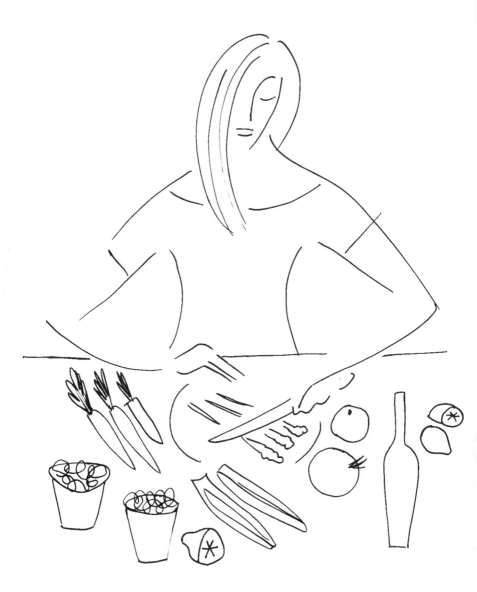

It's a real pity that in the minds of many slimmers, would-be slimmers, and even those simply worrying about a more healthy diet, food is seen as 'the enemy', and eating becomes a battleground. Such a battle is hard to win, because we're not sure who the enemy is, or what to do. Which foods are the 'goodies'? Which the 'baddies'? What will really work? Fasting? Food combining? One meal a day? And, of course, we're fighting a foe we really want to embrace (give in to the banquet, the binge), so determination is low. Perhaps, then, the answer is to get back to viewing food as part-pleasure, part-necessity, but never something against which to wage war. The aim of this chapter is to banish guilt and alter the see-saw of love and hate into something more balanced, via the facts and a large dose of common sense and reassurance.

you and your food

Q56

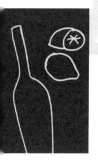

Calories are a measurement of energy, like the energy in food and that expended by humans. One kilocalorie (generally simply referred to as a calorie in nutrition, and certainly in this book) is the energy it takes to raise the temperature of one kilo of water by 1°C. For example, a food item containing 200 calories has enough energy to raise the temperature of 200kg of water by 1°C, or 2kg of water at 0°C to 100°C (boiling point). Human energy intake and output are also sometimes measured in kilojoules (now the official measure in the EU). One (kilo)calorie equals 4.2 kilojoules (kJ). A megajoule is 1,000 kilojoules.

Calories in food are measured by burning it in a calorimeter and measuring heat released into a surrounding water bath. Similarly, human energy output can be measured in a large form of the calorimeter – an airtight room where heat given off by the person is measured and converted into calories 'burnt'. By experiments like these we can measure the energy (calorie) cost of living and activity for anyone.

Q57

In what types of food are calories found?

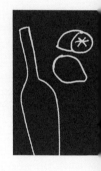

Almost everything that you eat or drink contains calories – with the notable exception of water. Some items, such as dried herbs, diet drinks and black tea (as examples), contain virtually no calories.

The four food groups that contain calories are carbohydrates, fat, protein (the 'macronutrients' – so called because they are the major nutrients) and alcohol. The food you eat can be made up from one or more of these food groups. Most foods contain at least two – e.g., a potato is mostly carbohydrate but also contains some fat and protein, and a beefsteak contains fat and protein but no carbs. Sugar is an exception – containing only carbohydrate – and pure oils are another exception – containing only fat.

The macronutrients each contain different quantities of calories. Carbohydrate contains 3.75 calories per gram, protein 4 and fat 9. Alcohol contains 7 calories per gram (most alcoholic drinks are a mixture of carbohydrate and alcohol).

Q58

What happens to food in the body?

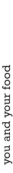

In the stomach, the gastric juices (mucus, hydrochloric acid and enzymes), aided by muscle contractions called peristalsis, break food down into semi-liquid chyme. Protein begins to be broken down into peptides. The only nutrients absorbed into the blood from the stomach are alcohol (why its effects are so quick), some simple sugars, water and water-soluble vitamins and minerals.

After up to 5 hours, the chyme is properly 'churned' and ready to move on. (Ingested liquids pass through the stomach quickly – sometimes in minutes. Carbohydrates pass through quickest – around 2 hours – protein next and fatty foods slowest.) Now the chyme gradually passes through the small intestine where it mixes with digestive juices and most nutrient absorption occurs.

Enzymes (proteins that speed bodily chemical reactions) finish the breakdown of protein into amino acids. Fats are broken down into glycerol and fatty acids; carbohydrates into maltose, glucose, fructose and galactose. Now these macronutrients, together with micronutrients (vitamins, minerals) and water, can pass

you and your food

through the intestinal walls and be carried by blood or lymph to where they are needed. This journey through the small intestine takes about 3 hours.

The simple sugars (the broken-down carbs) are carried by the blood to the liver. From there they can either be sent to the cells as glucose for energy, or converted into glycogen and stored in the liver or muscles, easily available when energy is required suddenly. Surplus is converted into fatty acids and stored in the adipose tissue.

The amino acids (broken-down protein) are also carried to the liver. From here they may used to build or repair muscle and enzymes. If extra energy is needed, the amino acids can be converted into a simple sugar and used as energy. Surplus amino acids can also be converted into fatty acids and stored in the adipose tissue.

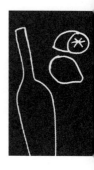

The fatty acids and glycerol (broken-down fat) are carried round the body as triglycerides in lymphatic fluid, and join the blood. When they find tissue needing energy, enzymes help it to be taken up. However, fat isn't normally the body's favourite energy source – glucose is (especially in the unfit). Unused blood fats are returned to the liver and then stored as adipose tissue. This can be converted back to energy when there's an energy deficit. Fat can't be converted to protein and only 5% of it (the glycerols) can be converted into glucose. However, dietary fat is more easily converted into body fat than either carbs or protein.

Back in the intestines, unabsorbed matter is passed through the large intestine, or colon, taking an average of 14 hours, where some of its water is absorbed, and then the remainder is finally excreted.

Q59

What happens in my body if I don't eat?

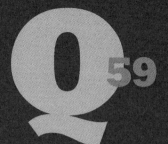

On water only, your body takes about 2 days to use up food eaten and glycogen stores. Blood sugar levels dip, leaving you weak, faint, dizzy and lacking concentration. You'll lose several pounds, mostly fluid, as you'll excrete extra urine. After 2 days, the body relies completely on its fat stores and lean tissue.

After 3 days, normally hunger pangs cease and bad breath begins, smelling like nail polish remover and due to ketones produced when fat is burnt in the absence of glucose. You'll feel the 'fasting high' – calm, full of energy and clear-headed. Metabolism slows to conserve energy and you may feel the cold more and be constipated. Loss of water – together with minerals, including sodium and potassium – continues. Weight loss is about 1 pound a day.

If the fast continues, it can strain both heart and kidneys. Nutrient deficiencies become apparent (e.g. without vitamin C, gums may bleed). Bone loss may occur and periods stop. Prolonged ketosis can be dangerous. Death from malnutrition and body malfunctions is likely within 60 days. See also Questions 70 and 88.

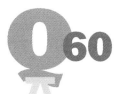 **60**

What happens if I eat more than I need?

More protein than needed can be converted into glucose for energy, if required, and then into body fat; excess carbs are converted into fat or nonessential amino acids; excess fat is stored as body fat. Alcohol can't be stored and must be eliminated (via breath or urine) or used for energy. Metabolism of alcohol takes precedence over carbs, so if you drink to excess, more carbs will store as fat. Excess calories of any type contribute to weight gain.

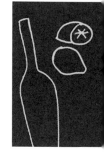

 **61**

What types of calories tend to put on most weight?

Surplus calories from all food types – fat, carbs and protein – have the potential to be stored as body fat. However, there's evidence that two types particularly help you gain weight if you overindulge. The first is fat (see Question 71). The second is simple carbs, such as sugar, white flour and all highly refined grain products like white bread, biscuits, cakes and all high-GI foods (see Question 66). In a 2004 study, rats fed a high-GI diet had 71% more body fat than those fed a low-GI diet, much of which was concentrated around their midriffs (see Question 47).

you and your food

Q62

Do carbohydrate foods encourage weight gain?

All foods eaten 'surplus to requirements' are stored as fat and that applies equally to surplus carbs. There may, however, be a small advantage in overeating complex carbs rather than fat, as fewer carb calories end up as body fat, because carbs burn about 25% of their calories turning into body fat, whereas dietary fat uses only about 3%. Thus, there'll be a little less fat gained from an excess carb intake of, say, 500 calories than a similar fat intake.

Carb consumption can, however, influence weight in other ways. For practical purposes, I am dividing carbs into two types. One is the simple and highly refined carbs, like table sugar, sweets and white flour; the other includes the complex and 'natural' carbs like pulses, wholegrains, fruits and vegetables. Simple carbs, like packet sugar and white flour, may be partly responsible for encouraging you to eat excess calories – for the following reasons:

1 They're often combined with fat in high-calorie ('junk') foods, like cakes, biscuits, pies, etc. These are likely to be 'binge' or 'comfort' foods. They usually 'slip down easily' and are eaten quickly, so full signals don't come into play in time to prevent eating excess.

2 Low-fat carbohydrate foods, like white bread, fatless cakes, slimmers' biscuits and desserts, and much confectionery don't make you feel full for long. They also cause blood sugar levels to rise rapidly and then dip rapidly (see Question 66), making you inclined to eat more.

On the other hand, the 'natural' carbs – like wholegrains (brown rice, oats, wholewheat pasta), roots and other starchy veg (like potatoes) and pulses, along with fresh fruits and vegetables – work in almost the opposite way. Being high in bulk and needing chewing, they slow down eating. They're not dense – so you get much more weight of food for your calories and it's hard to eat too much. They fill the stomach, take longer to digest, and stabilize blood-sugar levels – although some are less good at this than others (see Question 66). They are also less usually eaten with lots of fat. Many fruits and veg, pulses and oats, barley and rye are good sources of soluble fibre, which helps slow sugar absorption and lower blood LDL cholesterol.

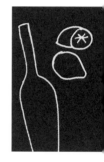

A diet high in carbs can increase fluid retention – they tend to 'soak up' more fluid; hence you may feel more bloated and your stomach look larger, but this isn't fat.

Researchers have pointed out that during the last world war the national diet was high in carbs (55%) and moderate in fat (33%), and the population was slimmer and healthier. The consensus seems to be that a diet high in 'natural' carbs doesn't encourage weight gain and is also 'good for you' in terms of nutrients, fibre and possible protection against disease, but that simple carbs can encourage weight gain especially around the midriff.

Is sugar so bad for you?

Dietary sugar can be divided into two categories. One is extrinsic – the types extracted from sugar cane or beet, honey, etc. and added to manufactured foods such as cakes, biscuits, desserts, confectionery or preserves, soft drinks and alcohol. The other is intrinsic – natural sugar found as part of the cellular structure of the plant, in foods such as fresh and dried fruit and vegetables. These fruits and veg make up an important and necessary part of a healthy diet and the sugar in them is more slowly absorbed, partly because of their soluble fibre content.

Extrinsic sugars can, as we saw in the previous question, lead to overeating, and the World Health Organization reported that a preference for sweet-fat mixtures has been observed in obese women and may be a factor in promoting excess energy consumption. Regular consumption of extrinsic sugar is a major cause of tooth decay. A high-sugar diet may promote insulin resistance, a condition where high blood sugar levels mean that the hormone insulin (which helps cells to absorb the glucose) is released in higher-than-normal amounts, and over a long period of time this may blunt the response of insulin, which then needs to be produced in ever greater quantities. Type-2 diabetics have insulin resistance. However, other types of simple carbohydrates can also promote high blood sugar levels (see Question 66). There is also some evidence that a high-sugar diet produces raised levels of a substance called glycosylated haemoglobin in the blood, high levels of which are associated with a greater risk of heart disease.

Sugar, in itself, contains no nutrients except calories. In addition, many commercially produced sugary foods are also low in nutrients (such as phytochemicals – plant compounds linked with good health) and fibre, and may be high in artificial additives and saturated or trans fats.

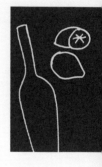

Although small amounts of sugary foods can be included in any weight-maintenance diet or even a slimming diet, some find it easier to avoid extrinsic sweet foods altogether and 're-educate' their taste. Brown sugar is not significantly nutritionally different from white sugar (and may be just coloured white sugar) and has a similar calorie value. Honey is also categorized as an extrinsic sugar. Containing more water, it has slightly fewer calories than sugar. Although good-quality natural honey is a well-known antiseptic, and may have other health benefits, most mass-produced honey is no better than sugar.

It's clear that extrinsic sugary foods do encourage surplus calorie consumption and contribute little, if anything, to the overall nutritional quality of your diet. So if you are trying to cut calories, such sugar calories, together with saturated fat calories, should be the first to go.

Q64

Intense artificial sweeteners such as aspartame, acesulfame-K and saccharin – used not only as tablet and granule sweeteners for drinks, cereals, etc. but also present in many commercial products, including diet drinks and many sweet diet products, are virtually calorie-free and, in theory, will help you to cut calories if you have a sweet tooth by replacing sugar in the diet.

However, in my opinion – and that of many experts – this isn't as useful long-term as it might seem, as replacing one sweetener with another does nothing to re-educate your palate to enjoy less sweet tastes. There is also some evidence from one UK study that people who have a high intake of artificial sweeteners actually take in more calories overall than people who don't. It is thought that the sweeteners may upset normal appetite mechanisms (or simply don't provide satiety value).

US research shows that, in animals, the sweetener aspartame hinders production of serotonin (the brain's 'happy hormone'), which can suppress appetite. Lack of it may be linked to depression and binge eating, and lab animals fed aspartame actually became obese.

There is always much debate about the safety of artificial sweeteners – for example, even those deemed safe by one government are banned by another. Some, such as saccharin and cyclamates, have been linked with cancer in lab animals and there seems to be little international consensus on their long-term safety. Aspartame (brand name Nutrasweet) shouldn't be used by children with a phenylketuronia defect.

Another sweetener is sorbitol. Related to sugar, it is a polyol (sugar alcohol) and is often used in diabetic products as it is absorbed less rapidly into the blood than sugar. Sorbitol is a little less sweet than sugar, but not calorie-free – it has 2.4 cals per gram (or 12 a teaspoonful) compared with 3.94 cals per gram (or 20 a teaspoonful) for sugar. In large amounts it can be laxative. Mannitol and xylitol are two similar polyol sweeteners.

Another sugar alternative is fructose – fruit sugar. This is not an 'artificial sweetener', as it is the sugar from fruit. Like sorbitol, it has a less marked effect on blood sugars. It contains about the same number of calories as sugar (sucrose) but is sweeter, so you need to use a little less. In large amounts, fructose may cause unwanted side effects. None of these sweeteners are necessary – even for diabetics – but may be useful for some.

So, should you use intense artificial sweeteners? Since we've been ingesting large amounts over the past 20 years or so, our collective weight has gone up, and sugar intake has hardly changed. There may be drawbacks and so there doesn't seem to be much point.

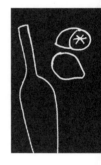

Q65

Although the most important factor in a weight-reducing diet is lowering total calorie content far enough to create an energy deficit (see Question 15), many international bodies with an interest in controlling obesity do encourage a diet rich in carbohydrates as a good way to lose weight and maintain the weight loss. However, the carbohydrate content of the diet needs to be mainly from natural or low GI or complex carbohydrates (see Questions 62 and 66), the fat content should be moderate or low, and overall calorie intake should be restricted.

The typical Western diet contains about 35–40% fat, 40–50% carbs and 15–20% protein. The US Department of Agriculture, in its recent paper on popular weight-loss diets (Jan 2001), says that 'low-fat diets containing a high proportion of complex carbohydrates, fruit and vegetables are naturally high in fiber and low in caloric density. Individuals consuming such diets consume fewer calories and lose weight.' The typical diet following these guidelines is, according to the USDA,

you and your food

96

25% fat, 60% carb and 15% protein, with a daily total energy intake of about 1,450 calories.

Indeed, in one trial, it was found that, over 14 days, moderate-fat, high-complex-carbohydrate reduction diets produce weight loss 'even when they are consumed ad libitum' (freely – i.e. calories weren't restricted). The most likely reason for this effect is that a high-complex-carb diet has a very high satiety value, so that a dieter has no inclination to overeat and can actually create a calorie deficit without feeling hungry. Such a diet will also naturally be high in insoluble and soluble fibre – incidentally, itself a complex carbohydrate. The World Health Organization, in a report, says fibre limits energy intake by lowering a food's density and allowing time for appetite-control signals to occur before large amounts of energy are consumed. Soluble fibre is particularly good at this.

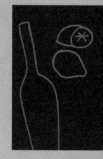

So the answer seems to be yes, this IS a very good way to diet and to maintain weight loss for many people. It is also one of the healthiest, because it will naturally reduce overall and saturated fat content of the diet, and should contain more than adequate amounts of fibre, most vitamins and minerals, and plant chemicals. It will also maintain healthy bowel function and avoid the constipation that is the plague of many low-calorie diets. However, it could be short on some nutrients (e.g. iron, if meat is avoided, or calcium, if high-fat dairy produce is avoided).

Q66

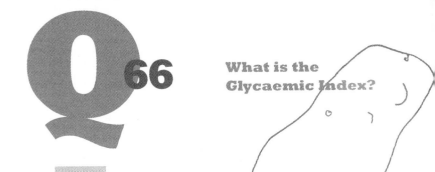

What is the Glycaemic Index?

Designed originally to help diabetics (it's important they control their blood-sugar levels), the Glycaemic Index shows the rate at which carbohydrate foods are absorbed into the bloodstream on a scale from 1 to 100. Glucose, which is absorbed most quickly, is rated 100.

The Glycaemic Index (GI) has relevance for those needing to follow a calorie-restricted diet, as foods with a low or moderate rating keep us full for longer, as well as steadying blood sugar levels, thus helping us feel less hungry and tired while dieting. Several recent research studies confirm that a low-GI diet is valuable in helping weight loss, weight maintenance and avoidance of an unhealthy 'apple shape' (see Question 47).

The lists opposite show some foods and their GI ratings, revealing some surprises. Not all foods high in fibre are low on the index, for one thing. Brown rice and wholemeal bread are high-GI foods, while yoghurt is low-GI. Also, the same food may have a different GI according to how it is cooked (e.g. boiled potatoes are medium, while mashed or baked are high) – even the variety (e.g.

basmati rice has a lower GI than white or brown).

Yoghurt and milk are low on the index because, although they contain simple sugars (lactose), the protein and fat content bring the overall GI down. Adding protein and/or fat to a high-GI food will make it have a lower 'GI effect' and slow absorption. So, for slimmers, high-GI carbs should be eaten with some protein or a little fat. Protein and fat foods are not measured on the GI, but they are both slowly absorbed into the bloodstream.

Measurements of GI vary according to how they were done, so I haven't given specific values for each food – but these lists give a reasonable consensus for common foods.

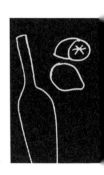

LOW-GI – 40 or less (slow-release, long-term energy – include plenty in your diet):
All pulses, including baked beans. • Barley, wholewheat pasta, whole rye grain. • Apples, dried apricots, peaches, cherries, grapefruit, plums, oranges, pears. • Avocados, courgettes, spinach, peppers, onions, mushrooms, leafy greens, leeks, green beans, broad beans, Brussels sprouts, mangetout, broccoli, cauliflower, tomatoes. • Yoghurt, milk, nuts.

MEDIUM-GI – 41–60 (medium-release, medium-term energy)
Sweet potatoes, boiled potatoes, raw carrots, sweetcorn, peas. • White pasta, oats, All Bran, noodles, popcorn. • Wholegrain rye bread, pitta bread, buckwheat, bulgar, white and brown basmati rice. • Grapes, kiwi fruit, mangoes, beetroot, figs, slightly under-ripe bananas.

HIGH-GI – over 60 (fast-release, short-term energy. For slimmers, best eaten along with protein/fat/low-GI foods)
Sugar, honey, pineapple, raisins, watermelon, ripe bananas.
• Baked/mashed potatoes, parsnips, cooked carrots, squash, swede.
• Brown/white rice other than basmati, rye crispbreads, wholemeal bread, white bread, rice cakes, couscous. • Cornflakes, Bran Flakes, instant oat cereal, puffed cereal, muffins. • Orange squash, dried dates.

you and your food

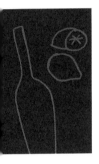

Carbohydrate foods that are low or moderate on the GI (see the previous question) are best as they are absorbed slowly into the bloodstream and keep blood sugar levels steady because they don't provoke a quick 'rush' of insulin.

Fresh fruits and vegetables are good, because they are relatively high in fibre and water and you get a lot of 'bulk' on your plate, which slows the rate of eating and allows the 'feeling full' mechanism to kick in before you eat too many calories. Foods especially high in soluble fibre are very good at keeping hunger at bay – examples are pulses, mangoes, dried apricots, Brussels sprouts, peas and spring greens.

Moderate amounts of fat and lean protein, both of which take longer to be absorbed into the blood than carbs, will help keep you feeling full for longer. This is probably one reason why most people are not successful long-term on diets that are very, very low in fat. You need some fat to keep you satisfied!

you and your food

100

Q68

How can I avoid feeling weak, tired and dizzy on a slimming diet?

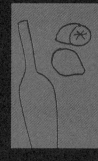

You need to eat regularly – having, say, three smallish meals and two small snacks a day, including low-GI foods (see Question 66). This will help keep your blood sugar levels steady. Weakness and dizziness are possible symptoms of low blood sugar. What happens then is that you're inclined to eat something high in simple sugars, e.g. biscuits, and, while this raises blood sugar quickly, it will also dip quickly, leaving you feeling even worse.

Ideal snacks to keep blood sugar even are a small handful of nuts and dried apricots, an apple and a few cherries, or a pot of low-fat yoghurt. Ideal lunches and suppers are basmati rice or new potatoes with plenty of fresh vegetables or salad and chicken, fish or lean meat.

Tiredness may or may not be a symptom of unsuitable low-calorie dieting. If you've only become tired since starting a diet, you should ensure it contains enough of the essential nutrients, including iron, B vitamins, vitamin C, etc. Perhaps you're trying to lose weight on too few calories – increase them slightly and you may feel better. If none of this applies, see your doctor.

Do I need to feel hunger pangs in order to lose weight?

Not really. Hunger pangs are the normal stomach muscle contractions which help to 'mash up' food when you eat it (see Question 58). When your stomach is empty, however, the contractions have nothing to do except churn up air – and this is the noise and sensation of 'pangs' you feel. At this stage your brain may also be quietly telling you that you need to eat because it is receiving signals from your body to that effect.

Obviously, if you follow a diet very low in calories, which involves eating fewer meals, or meals of the types of food that get quickly digested by your stomach and are low in bulk (like many of the typical ready-meals for dieters), then you will feel hunger pangs. This is a classic diet pattern that many slimmers have followed down the years but, as you will see if you read elsewhere in this section, this isn't a brilliant way to slim at all.

If you eat a diet reduced moderately in calories to no lower than your BMR requirements, that is high in natural and complex carbohydrates, including plenty of fresh veg and fruit and items low on the GI (see Question 66),

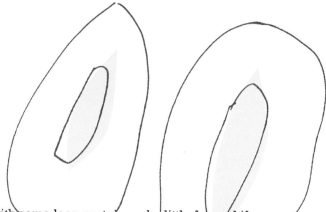

with some lean protein and a little fat, and if you eat three times a day plus two between-meal snacks, then you can lose weight without ever feeling a proper hunger pang. You literally 'fool' the body into feeling full. One study showed that the average slimmer can cut calories by 450 a day on this type of diet without feeling hunger pangs, and this would be enough to lose nearly 1lb a week in weight. This type of diet is explained in more detail elsewhere in the section.

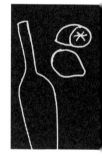

As the answer to Question 65 explained, people who followed such a diet in one experiment actually didn't have to count calories at all – they ate all they wanted of the allowed foods every day and still lost weight! Taking extra exercise will also burn off calories and allow you to eat more – studies show that for most people, exercise doesn't increase hunger.

To sum up, diets that make you hungry are not going to help you succeed. (Interestingly, when people go on a total fast, they say that their hunger pangs disappear within three days or so – but that's a different story!)

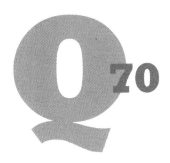

Does a high-protein diet have any special benefits for getting or keeping me slim?

A diet high in protein (30% or more of total calories) will only help you lose weight if the other macronutrients – carbohydrates, alcohol and fat – are reduced sufficiently to create an overall calorie deficit. It's this deficit that matters more than any combination – or exclusion – of nutrients.

Most high-protein diets are actually reduced-calorie diets containing a high proportion of protein, a very-low proportion of carbohydrate (sometimes almost none) and varying amounts of fat – sometimes a lot. However, a high-protein, very-low-carbohydrate diet does have properties that can make it seem easier to lose weight.

Initial weight loss will usually be high as, with a low-carb intake, the body's carb stores (glycogen) are depleted, and with them water. Also the very low carb and fibre content will naturally tend to reduce retained fluid. Water loss, of course, isn't fat loss and, once the low-carb diet is abandoned, weight lost through fluid will return.

It's also been reported that a high-protein diet can increase dietary induced thermogenesis (DIT) – meaning it may help your metabolism speed up and thus create a

you and your food

104

greater calorie deficit than would be apparent with other types of diet. One estimate is that this could account for burning 25% of the calories in a protein meal.

Lastly, a very-low-carb, high-protein diet produces ketones in the blood that are responsible for reducing appetite. Also many high-protein foods, like eggs and lean meat, contain the amino acid leucine, which helps control hunger and burn fat. This makes such a diet relatively easy to stick to and could explain why many find it easy to lose weight on such a diet.

Sadly, however, as with many things that seem too good to be true, there is a downside. High intake of protein – particularly animal protein – is associated with various health problems. It can lead to excessive production of waste products – particularly urea – and strain the kidneys (increasing the likelihood of stones) and liver. Increased levels of uric acid in the blood can increase the risk of gout. High protein intake is also linked with bone demineralization and may exacerbate osteoporosis.

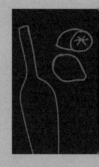

There's also some evidence linking a high protein intake with high blood pressure. Constipation can result, as the diet is low in fibre, and bad breath is a side effect of protein-induced ketosis. High-protein diets may also be high in saturated fat, linked with many health problems. A high-protein, low-carb diet can also result in a shortfall of various important nutrients.

A calorie-reduced, high-protein diet may therefore help you lose weight but isn't healthy and isn't recommended. The diet as outlined in Question 65 will also stave off hunger and produce weight loss, while being healthy.

you and your food

Q71

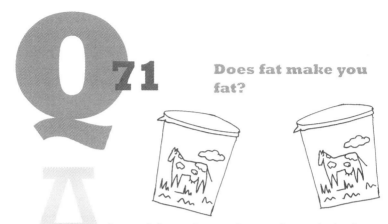

Does fat make you fat?

Excess of any of the major nutrients – fat, carbohydrate or even protein – can make you fat. However, some diets (many high-protein, low carb ones) actually have a high fat content. So you can lose weight on fat. However, such diets work because they're self-limiting – you can only eat so much fat and protein without carbohydrate.

Having said that, one of the most effective ways to keep weight down is to reduce fat intake. One recent study of obese people found their fat intake was far higher and carb intake far lower than recommended levels, and concluded that 'dietary intake, especially fat intake, seems to be the main factor contributing to obesity...' A 1998 trial found 'significant positive correlations... between the percentage of dietary energy as total fat, and body fatness...' An overview of trials on 1,728 individuals in 2000 concluded 'a reduction in dietary fat without restriction of total energy intake prevents weight gain in subjects of normal weight...' So, according to that last research, by reducing fat intake you can eat unrestricted calories and not put on weight!

But why does fat make you fat? As we saw in Question 62, dietary fat is very efficient at storing itself as body fat (about 97%), unlike carbs and protein. And, of all the nutrients, fat is the most energy-dense at 9 cals/gram (carbs are 3.75 and protein 4). Fat is also very palatable, especially combined with sugar or salt. It has good mouth-feel and 'slips down easily'. For this reason, and being cheap, it is a key ingredient in many commercial products that are easy to overeat. Research shows that high-fat, low-bulk foods (like chocolate or cheese) can make us eat to excess before the brain signals we're full.

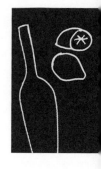

The fat element of the diet can be taken away with no perceived difference in satiety. A recent study found it was possible to remove 450 calories' worth of fat from the average high-fat main meal without it being noticed – enough to produce a weekly weight loss of nearly 1lb. Research shows that by reducing the fat content of meals, but keeping their overall bulk (via plenty of natural and complex carbohydrates and lean protein), people don't feel hungry and don't overeat. As the WHO says in its 2001 report on obesity, fat appears to be the key macronutrient that undermines the body's weight-regulatory system.

Yet there is an exception that proves the rule. More and more evidence is being gathered that one type of fat – the omega-3s found in oily fish, some plants and other produce (see Question 72) – may actually be less 'fattening' than other fats and have a beneficial effect on metabolism and insulin sensitivity. So it's wise to cut right back on saturates, trans fats and (to a certain extent) omega-6 fats, while ensuring adequate omega-3s.

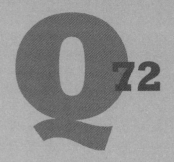

Q72 What are the different types of fat and which are good and which bad for you?

Fats to cut back on...

SATURATED FATS: fats solid at room temperature are highest in saturates. Examples of foods high in saturates: fat in meat and dairy products, and many commercial bakes. A diet high in saturates can raise LDL blood cholesterol and 'block' the work of the essential fatty acids (opposite). Most of us eat much more than needed – in a healthy reduced-fat diet you need no more than 5% of calories from saturates.

TRANS FATS: unsaturated fats hardened (or hydrogenated) in the manufacture of commercial foods like margarine. They are nutritionally similar to saturated fats, or worse, as they raise blood LDL cholesterol and may also lower 'good' HDL cholesterol. They are best avoided.

POLYUNSATURATED FATS USED IN COOKING: highly unsaturated fats, which are liquid even when kept in the fridge (such as corn, sunflower and safflower oil and blended vegetable oils) are best avoided in high-temperature cooking as this can cause oxidation and the production of free radicals and may be linked to increased risk of cancer.

you and your food

108

Fats to eat in moderation...

POLYUNSATURATES, COLD OR AT LOW TEMPERATURE:
Polyunsaturates are found in high quantities in most
vegetable and seed oils (which are rich sources of the
omega-6 group of fats including the essential fatty acid
linoleic acid). While we need this fat in our diet, most of
us eat more than we need of the omega-6 group.

Instead, we should try to eat more of the polyunsaturates
that contain high levels of the omega-3 group of fats,
including the essential fatty acid alpha-linolenic acid. This
group is found primarily in oily fish and in linseeds
(flaxseeds), hemp, groundnut oil, rapeseed oil, pumpkin
seeds and oil, walnuts and walnut oil, and – surprisingly -
dark leafy greens are a fair source.

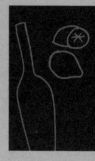

Regular intake of the omega-6 and omega-3 essential fats
is important for growth, body maintenance and health. Oily
fish contains two special omega-3 fats – EPA and DHA –
which are particularly good for health protection.

In general, the polyunsaturated group tend to lower
blood LDL cholesterol but don't raise 'good' HDL.

Aim for a diet with around 10% of total calories as
polyunsaturates and a 2:1 ratio omega-6 to omega-3.
Store oils in cool dark conditions and use within weeks
to prevent oxidation.

MONOUNSATURATES: tend to be liquid at room temperature
and solid when cooled. Foods high in monounsaturates
include olive oil, rapeseed oil, most nuts, and avocados.
Monounsaturates are healthy as they may lower LDL
cholesterol and raise HDL. They are also better for
cooking, as they tend not to oxidize under heat

Q73

As we saw in Question 71, fat tends to keep you fat, and the opposite seems true – reduced-fat eating can keep you slim. The World Health Organization, having viewed all the evidence, says modest energy-deficit diets (i.e. not crash) and 'ad libitum' (eat freely) low-fat diets appear to have a better long-term outcome than very-low-cal diets. They also say that low-fat, high-carb diets are superior in maintaining weight loss 2 years on, compared with standard calorie-counting diets. However, this review was published before a barrage of evidence emerged on the benefits of a low-GI diet (see Question 66) for slimming.

Any diet which produces long-term weight loss in obese or very overweight people will probably bring health benefits, because overweight is linked with so many health problems, and a moderate low-fat diet with a high intake of complex carbs, fruit and veg, and adequate lean protein is probably healthier than other types of calorie-reducing diet. Such diets have been shown to lower blood pressure and 'bad' LDL blood cholesterol, and may have a small effect in lowering risk of heart disease.

However, there are very healthy fat-reduced diets and less healthy low-fat diets. The difference is in the amounts and types of fat allowed in any reduced-fat regime. Very low-fat diets may actually increase the risk of heart disease. In 2005, researchers at Washington University discovered that zero-fat diets can stop you burning up sugar, cholesterol and other fats from your bloodstream, and can even cause liver failure. Not all fat is bad! A good slimming diet (such as most low-GI diets and some others) reduces the level of saturated and trans fats to a minimum, while retaining adequate amounts of the essential omega-3s and, to a lesser extent, omega-6s in the diet.

These EFAs have been shown to be vital in maintaining good health and helping prevent disease. They can lower LDL cholesterol and raise 'good' HDL, lower blood pressure, balance the immune system, help prevent stroke, improve brain function, improve arthritis pain, help lift depression, and more.

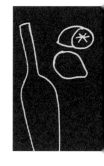

To provide adequate essential fats, your low-fat diet should go no lower than 20–25% fat and, for omega-3s, should incorporate regular oily fish (2 portions a week), nuts, pumpkin, flax and other seeds, leafy greens and oils from these items. People who dislike many of these, should take a daily fish oil supplement rich in omega-3s. Such a diet will also supply adequate omega-6s.

These EFAs are better absorbed when saturated and trans fat intake is low. Small amounts of olive oil can also be used, as monounsaturates help prevent colon cancer, may raise HDL cholesterol levels and appear to have none of the negative effects of trans and saturated fats.

What exactly is food combining and is it a good system for weight loss?

A

Invented over 70 years ago by US doctor William Hay, this involves separating intake of carbohydrates (e.g. bread and potatoes) and proteins (like meat and dairy produce), so you never mix the two at the same meal. The theory is, basically, nonsense.

However, the system also emphasizes whole fresh foods, and avoids refined foods. The overall content is thus probably healthier than the average Western diet, but lack of protein with carbohydrate meals can result in low blood sugar. Weight loss will almost certainly follow for anyone who is overweight and sticks to the regime. There's no 'magic' in the food combining aspect, though, to produce weight loss – it is simply the result of creating a calorie deficit. It's hard to eat a lot of calories on a diet that places so many restrictions upon how, when and what you eat. (Try unlimited pasta with no meat or egg sauce!)

There are easier ways to eat a healthy, slimming diet – why replace one set of eating fads with another? No doubt proponents will argue the point.

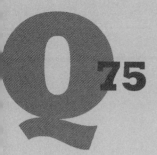

Q75

Is eating nothing but raw food a good dieting idea?

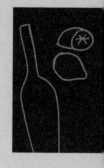

A raw-food diet tends to consist almost exclusively of plant foods – vegetables, fruit, nuts and seeds. You could also eat some raw fish or meat, but raw-eaters tend to be vegan.

Because a raw diet is so high in such items, it has a very low calorie-to-bulk ratio – meaning you get lots to chew on for very few calories. It's almost impossible to eat too many calories on such a regime so you would lose weight quite rapidly. Also, hunger isn't nearly as much of a problem as you'd think, as the very high fibre content tends to slow the rate of eating and helps the body's satiety mechanism.

However, a raw-only diet isn't such a good idea as it seems. It usually means a huge change in diet habits, and research shows most people can't sustain radical diet changes. Also, it isn't varied or balanced (protein and starch content are low) and could lead to dietary deficiencies. Lastly, rapid weight loss isn't such a good idea; most studies show weight lost slowly is much more likely to stay off.

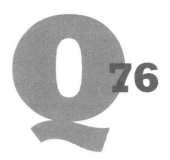

Q76

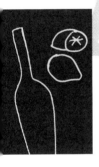

Eating plenty of fruit and veg should help your weight-loss campaign, for various reasons. One, they all contain a high ratio of bulk to calories. This is because of their high water and, generally, low fat content. For example, apples are 88% water and carrots 90%. Two, they offer plenty of 'bite'. Because of their high cellulose/fibre content they help you feel full, even though they contain few calories. Raw or lightly cooked fruit and veg also provides 'crunch' factor. Because of these effects, it's been shown that, while an average 125g apple takes around 3 minutes to eat and contains just 60 calories or so, a small 25g chocolate bar containing 130 calories takes just 1 minute. As we've seen in previous questions, slow eating helps weight control and helps you feel more satisfied.

Fresh and dried fruits are natural sources of sweetness, and make good substitutes for sweets and chocolate. Also, many fruits and vegetables are low on the Glycaemic Index (see Question 66), with plenty of soluble fibre, and help you feel full for longer and keep blood sugar levels even.

you and your food

114

Q77

Is regular snacking between meals a good or bad idea?

Regular high-fat and/or high-sugar snacks, like crisps, pastries, etc. are not a good idea. Apart from supplying many extra calories and grams of fat, research shows people tend to snack on these when they aren't hungry. This urge can be controlled by a diet rich in foods low on the Glycaemic Index (see Question 66). However, healthy between-meal snacks can be excellent when trying to control calorie intake as they help keep blood sugar constant, keep hunger at bay for few calories and help avoid snacking on less favourable fare.

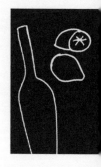

Ideal snacks are low-GI and low in calories and fat, like apples, dried apricots, raw veg, natural low-fat yoghurt or a couple of spoonfuls of brown basmati rice. Even nuts and seeds can be eaten in moderation – one study found that between-meal snacking on peanuts, almonds or peanut butter didn't result in weight gain as satiety value was high and participants automatically adjusted calorie intake. Other research shows frequent eating helps people regulate energy intake. Between-meal snacks should, however, be small if trying to lose weight.

you and your food

115

Q78

How many meals should I eat a day for optimum weight loss and is there any basis for the idea of dieting on just one meal a day?

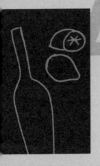

The consensus of opinion is that you should eat small, regular meals. Eating regularly helps keep blood sugar levels even, keeps you feeling full, helps you cope better psychologically with eating fewer calories and helps avoid bingeing.

Most who try one meal a day can only manage it for a short time – psychologically, physically and socially it doesn't suit us. Blood sugar levels are usually low for much of the day apart from the few hours after the meal, resulting in fatigue, dizziness, poor concentration, etc. Also, the tendency is to pile much more food on your plate than normal – research shows the more you put on your plate, the more you eat. The willpower needed is tremendous, and unplanned bingeing probable. A single meal, followed by what is effectively a mini-fast for the rest of the day, may result in a drop in levels of the thyroid hormone T3, which otherwise helps raise metabolic rate. Although calories are likely to be restricted naturally (you can only eat so much at one sitting) there are other, easier and healthier, ways of slimming.

you and your food

116

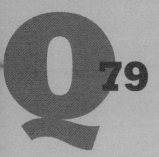

How important is breakfast in a good slimming campaign?

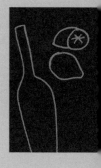

Studies indicate that people who eat breakfast tend to be slimmer and have lower overall fat intake, lower calorie intake and higher carb intake than those who don't. Indeed, a recent study revealed that people who eat most of their food earlier in the day consume significantly fewer calories than people who like to eat in the evening.

But the debate is still open. It's true there are lots of overweight people who eat breakfast. However, the answers to previous questions show that regular eating is a key to successful weight loss, and of all the meals, breakfast is the one it makes most sense not to skip.

This is because you've 'fasted' all night and blood-sugar levels are low. If you skip breakfast, you'll find it harder to resist sweet and fatty 'junk' snacks later in the morning. If you have a breakfast containing some complex (preferably low-GI) carbohydrate, some protein and a little fat, you'll be unlikely to do this. You should get everything you need in a breakfast containing no more than 20% of your total day's calories. If you prefer a larger breakfast, have a smaller lunch and/or evening meal.

you and your food

Does food eaten late convert straight to body fat while you sleep?

This really is one of those old wives' tales that sticks and sticks! As we saw in Question 58, most of the food you eat takes a few hours to be broken down and absorbed before it can even begin to be used by the body for energy, or stored as fat. The next fact to remember is that we continue to burn calories even while we are asleep – quite a few of them. An average person may burn, say, 60 calories an hour for their basal metabolic rate (which is the rate you're burning calories when you are asleep). So, suppose you have your evening meal at 8 pm, by 8 am the next morning, you will have burnt up 12 x 60, or 720 calories, just lying there asleep or reading or whatever. (Indeed, one recent study found that feeding people a large meal in the evening increased their metabolic rate for several hours after the meal even as they slept.) Unless your evening meal contained more calories than that, then there won't have been any spare to be laid down as fat.

Even if food is converted into body fat, once you create a small energy deficit, by exercising or by taking

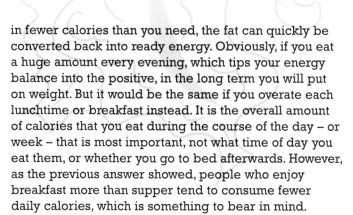

in fewer calories than you need, the fat can quickly be converted back into ready energy. Obviously, if you eat a huge amount every evening, which tips your energy balance into the positive, in the long term you will put on weight. But it would be the same if you overate each lunchtime or breakfast instead. It is the overall amount of calories that you eat during the course of the day – or week – that is most important, not what time of day you eat them, or whether you go to bed afterwards. However, as the previous answer showed, people who enjoy breakfast more than supper tend to consume fewer daily calories, which is something to bear in mind.

Few people manage to balance their energy input and output exactly – eating only just exactly enough at each meal and no more to compensate precisely for the amount of calories they've burnt up since the last meal – or are going to burn up before the next meal. Who could be so clever – or would want to be so obsessive? Energy balancing is a long-term process, not a short-term thing.

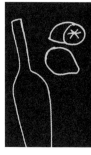

you and your food

Q81

What are the best drinks to choose on a slimming diet, and why?

Boring as this may sound, plain water really is the ideal drink for a weight-watcher. This is because water is calorie-free, contains no artificial additives, hydrates you and can even help to fill you up – a glass before a meal and one sipped during a meal will help to blunt the appetite a little. You could also go for water with a dash of real fruit juice added, for an exciting change.

Now, here is some good news. For something hot, experts have decided that it is, after all, OK to choose tea. The latest trial results, revealed at the American College of Cardiology Conference in 2001, show that tea really is good for the cardiovascular system. It can help to prevent blood clots and open up the arteries in people with severe heart disease. It is also rich in antioxidants, which can also help prevent heart disease and perhaps cancers. Moreover, it is virtually calorie-free and, at 40mg caffeine for an average 200ml (7fl oz) serving, you could have 7 cups a day before getting near the recommended maximum caffeine intake of 300mg a day.

It has often been said that tea is diuretic and that it

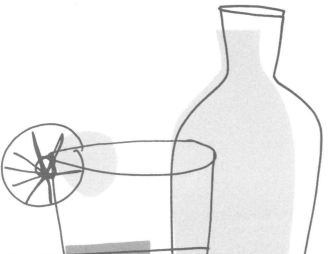

doesn't count towards the day's fluid intake. In fact, tea is only mildly diuretic and will only increase urine excretion by a small amount – nowhere near enough to cancel out the amount of liquid you ingest. One drawback: tea shouldn't be drunk with food, as it can hinder the absorption of minerals.

Green tea and redbush (roibosch) tea are both virtually calorie-free and contain antioxidants while being low in caffeine or actually caffeine-free, so they are both excellent drinks too. Redbush tea tastes similar to ordinary black tea. Herbal teas, such as rosehip, camomile or peppermint, are all low in calories at between 2 and 12 a cup, and are pleasant to drink (if you like them). Some may have mild health properties too (e.g. camomile will help you sleep, peppermint may aid digestion).

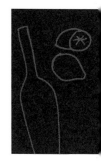

you and your food

Q82

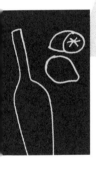

That's what this book aims to help with. Questions 32, 61–71 and 73 give the background to what makes an ideal slimming diet. Question 83 discusses the 'perfect' diet and Question 85 tells you how many calories you should be slimming on. From this you can build a picture of sensible and successful dieting. Question 84 also reviews what I judge to be the 5 best diets, where all the pros and cons of each are listed. From this you can make a choice. Alternatively, you can use the information in this book to choose or build your own diet.

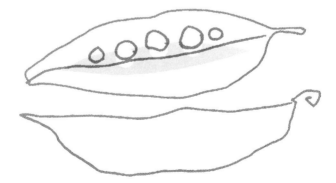

Is there such as thing as 'the perfect diet'?

It's the one that gets you slim without pain, keeps you at your maintenance weight without pain – and that you like. Of course, that will vary from person to person, but various bodies decree the ideal diet is one that:

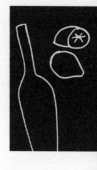

- Reduces weight at slow or moderate speed.
- Is moderately low in fat and high in carbohydrate.
- Is low in density and high in bulk – meaning lots of veg and fruit, as well as enough starch and lean protein.
- Offers high chance of compliance – i.e. you'll stick to it. The consensus seems to be this will be a diet offering high satiety value, presenting plenty on the plate and that isn't difficult to follow. The reduced-fat, low-saturates, high-complex-carb, low-GI diet wins on all counts – and it is healthy.

As far as weight maintenance goes, again, the reduced-fat, high-complex-carb diet wins. The World Health Organization reports that such a diet has been shown to be superior to a calorie-counting diet for maintaining weight two years later. Both for weight loss and for weight maintenance, regular exercise is a vital element.

Q84

What are the most popular diets and how do they compare?

The following diet types I consider the most popular and/or famous. My star ratings (out of five) are based on ease, effectiveness, cost, palatability, satiety and healthiness.

Glycaemic index diets *****
The basis of diets such as *The Glucose Revolution* is that a diet containing most of its carbs as foods with a low or moderately low GI (see Question 66) will help keep blood sugar levels even and hunger pangs at bay. These are among the best healthy all-round diets for slimmers.

Calorie-counting diets ****
This involves deciding on a suitable daily calorie intake, with the help of a guide to the calorie content of foods or calorie-counted menus. Most foods must be measured and common sense used to provide a healthy balanced diet.

Low-fat diets ****
These aim to reduce total fat (the most calorie-dense nutrient) and usually concentrate on getting saturates as low as possible, while essential polyunsaturated fats

(and/or monounsaturated fats) are allowed in small quantities. *Patrick Holford's Fat Burner Diet* is a low-fat regime, as is *The F-Plan* and most GI diets. Aim for a low-fat diet containing around 20–25% total fat. Diets lower than 20% fat are described as 'very low fat' and are not good either health-wise or for compliancy.

High-fibre diets ****
The F-Plan (Audrey Eyton 1982) was the first, and probably is still the best, high-fibre diet. The theory is that a high intake of fibre quickly fills you up and also keeps hunger pangs at bay between meals. Slightly different from a low-GI diet as some high-fibre foods aren't necessarily low-GI.

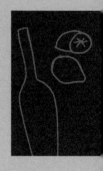

Meal replacements ***
You swap one or two meals a day for the meal replacement – usually a drink – which is calorie-counted and nutrition-balanced. Because of its ease and the fact it takes away much decision making, many people find it successful. The most well known make is probably SlimFast.

High-protein diets **
Diets containing high levels of protein and low levels of carbs work by either reducing total calorie intake and/or increasing metabolic rate and the rate at which fat can be burnt off. Most contain high levels of fat (e.g. *Atkins Diet Revolution*) while others, such as the *South Beach Diet*, are lower in fat content. Many medics believe a high protein, high saturates diet may be dangerous to health long term.

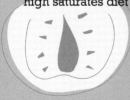

How many calories a day do most people need to reduce to in order to lose weight?

The larger a daily energy deficit you create (see Question 15) the more weight you will lose, but you could create a tiny (say 50 cals/day) deficit and lose it very slowly over time. The pros of a large deficit are rapid weight loss and the cons are hunger, nutrient deficiency and non-compliance. The pros of very slow weight loss are good compliance and higher nutrient intake, but few results – a compromise seems best.

Some experts recommend dieting at basal metabolic rate (BMR, see Question 2). Then whatever activity you do on top of this creates your calorie deficit – the more you do, the quicker you lose weight.

The World Health Organization says the lowest calorie limit for dieting (not under medical supervision) should be 1,200/day, but that most people tolerate best a daily deficit of between 500–600 calories. From my experience of helping people lose weight, this is right. It will result in a weekly weight loss of a pound or a little more, which equals about 4 stones a year! This is also the level linked with your best chance of maintaining weight loss.

For most people, a daily deficit of 500–600 calories will not take them as low as just 1,200 cals. The US Department of Agriculture says that even in the absence of physical activity, diets of 1,400–1,500 cals/day result in weight loss for adults, so you may not need to go as low as 1,200–1,500 cals/day. If you're very overweight, very tall, young, etc., and have a high metabolic rate, you'll need perhaps 2,000 cals/day at least, at first. Go too low, you'll feel hungry and deprived and won't stick to the diet. On the other hand, if you have a very low metabolic rate you may need to go a little lower than 1,400–1,500 to achieve 1lb a week loss. You may decide to increase activity levels to raise your energy output.

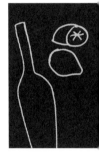

Lastly, if you decide to diet on the same level as your BMR, then eat that many calories a day. If you don't want to count calories, various plans do this for you, or see Question 93.

While dieting, recheck your metabolic rate, as losing weight lowers BMR and you may need to lower calorie intake slightly. Also remember that exercise will help raise total energy output and let you eat more, or lose weight a little quicker. It will also conserve muscle, which helps minimize the metabolic slowing due to dieting.

Q86 What exactly is a crash diet?

A diet very low in calories (usually anything less than 1,000 calories a day) is described as a 'crash diet', often with a 'faddy' eating element to it – for example, nothing but eggs and milk, or cheese and tomatoes – which will result in rapid weight loss. Usually over 3lb (1.5kg) a week is promised.

Q87 Are crash diets really such a bad idea?

Amongst health experts, crash diets are seen as a bad idea for most people as:

1 They encourage loss of more lean tissue (muscle) than diets which produce a slower weight loss on a higher calorie level.

2 They may be lacking in nutrients – both macronutrients such as fat, protein or carbohydrate, and micronutrients such as vitamins and minerals.

3 They don't encourage sensible eating habits and this means that after the crash diet is over weight is easily regained. In time, this can turn into a 'yo-yo' dieting habit, which is very demoralizing.

Q 88

Is fasting a good idea for weight loss – and how long can I fast?

In Question 59 there's a detailed explanation of what happens to your body when you don't eat. After reading it, you will probably agree that fasting as a means of long-term weight loss isn't such a good idea, even though it's bound to produce good results while it lasts.

There are many advocates of fasting, and it is a well-recognized way of life in India. There are, however, inherent dangers in fasting and, once the fast is over, the almost inevitable regaining of weight (see the previous question), so it does seem rather pointless.

Having said all that, some people enjoy short regular periods of fasting – say, one day a week, or a two-day fast once a month, or a week's fast four times a year – and are none the worse for it. Used in such a way, it is possible that fasting might help keep weight stable. However, for most people, I am sure that a good detox diet is a better idea; see Question 191.

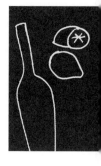

you and your food

Q89

What's the least number of calories I can eat to slim and stay healthy long-term?

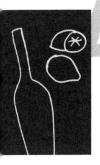

The World Health Organization says the lowest recommended dieting level (except under medical supervision) is 1,200 calories a day, but prefers 1,400–1,500. One good rule is that you shouldn't diet below your own basal metabolic rate – the rate at which your body uses calories doing nothing. Average BMR for women is around 1,500 calories a day.

You'd then lose weight according to calories burned in your daily activity over and above BMR. For very sedentary people this is as low as a few hundred; for active people it can be double BMR – and for them I would say dieting on the BMR would actually be too low. However, very active people rarely need to diet.

Another good rule is to increase calorie intake if weight loss goes over the sensible 1–2lb a week dietitians recommend. You needn't worry about counting calorie intake as long as sensible weight loss is proceeding. This also holds true of weight maintenance – you needn't count calories for life; just weigh yourself occasionally to ensure nothing's changed.

Q90

What are the pros and cons of very-low-cal, liquid-only diets?

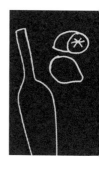

VLCDs, as they're called, are mostly used to get weight off severely overweight people under medical supervision, before operations or when their life is endangered. They're also sold as slimming aids to the public.

Each meal is usually around 250 calories and, on such a regime (3 a day in total), weight loss is rapid. If only replacing one or two meals a day, results are slower. The meals are fortified with vitamins, minerals and so on, and should be nutritionally balanced.

Some people find it easier to replace a meal with a formula, as the worry about what to eat is removed – as is room for temptation and/or cheating.

Disadvantages could be that you've little choice and the regime can be very dispiriting. These formulas do nothing to re-educate you to better eating habits, lean tissue loss may be greater than on a higher-calorie regime and, once off the system, weight may return. The WHO says VLCDs by individuals without medical supervision is unwise and shouldn't be recommended. However, replacing one meal a day can be useful.

you and your food

131

Q91

Can you really block calories in food so that they're not absorbed?

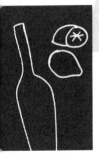

The prescription slimming pill Xenical works on this principle – blocking the breakdown of dietary fat in the intestines, with the result that about 30% passes through unabsorbed. The fat substitute 'food' Olestra is virtually calorie-free because of a similar principle. It is only used in a few food products in the US and has not been approved in the UK. Both Olestra and Xenical may have unwanted side effects, such as diarrhoea and flatulence, if anything other than a low-fat diet is followed, and the fat-soluble vitamins are also passed through the body, which could lead to mineral deficiencies.

Over-the-counter or mail-order pills called 'starch blockers' have been on sale for years, claiming to block the starch in your food. These claims are, by and large, unproven and, in any case, within a healthy diet it wouldn't be desirable to block starch. Fat-blocking pills, often called 'fat magnets', again are of very limited, if any, use. They may block a few calories from each meal but the overall amount is too little to make any real difference to the average diet.

Q 92

Is it true there are foods that contain 'negative calories'?

The idea goes that foods such as celery, cabbage, beansprouts and so on are so low in calories and high in fibre that your digestive system burns more calories digesting them than the foods actually contain, thereby creating a calorie deficit.

As with many such ideas, it does contain a grain of truth – some foods (mostly vegetables) are very low in calories. Also, as we've seen in Question 2, when you eat, your metabolic rate speeds up via dietary induced thermogenesis (DIT). With some foods, DIT can be quite high – but the highest producers of DIT are protein foods, burning up to 25% of their calories during digestion. Sadly, all protein foods contain reasonable amounts of calories, so even allowing for this effect, you're still in a positive energy situation!

The vegetables mentioned above don't create a deficit, even though it would be almost impossible to get fat on them. To eat enough celery (at 7 cals/100g) to get an average day's intake of about 2,000 calories, you would have to eat 28.5 kilos!

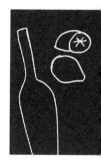

Q93

Can I lose weight without drastic diet changes or calorie counting?

If you've been eating a diet high in fat and calories that has made you overweight, the healthiest way to slim is to cut the fat right back, in which case, research shows you can eat carbs fairly freely. Such a diet would, however, sometimes entail weighing or measuring items, or at least reading the nutrition panels on packs, and the carb element should be healthy 'complex carbs', like wholegrains and pasta, fruit and vegetables. This has been shown to be the easiest and most successful way of slimming for many people long-term.

If you've a sweet tooth or like 'junk food', then eating this way will obviously mean drastic changes to your diet. The only way to avoid this is to eat what you want, but in smaller amounts. This is calorie counting by another name – you don't look items up or measure them, but just eat two-thirds or half of what you would normally. The disadvantages of this are that you may feel hungry and it doesn't re-educate your palate to enjoy healthier foods. You'd increase your chances of success by adding plenty of extra low-cal vegetables and salads to help fill you up.

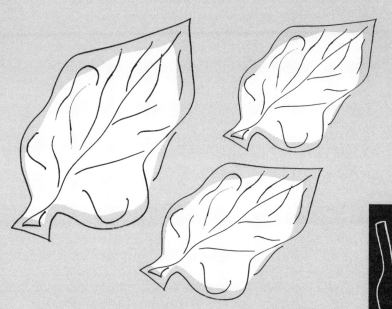

The last idea you could try is to increase the exercise you do. If you burn an extra few hundred calories a day (say, an hour's cycling), then, in theory, you could lose weight without changing eating habits at all. In practice, it is best to combine exercise with a moderately reduced-calorie, reduced-fat diet.

One experiment proved most overweight people can cut the calories in an average main course by 450 without even noticing! That would result in a weekly weight loss of nearly 1lb without doing another thing. Sadly (or gladly), weight control in the long term IS mostly about eating in a healthier way for the rest of your life – and taking more exercise.

Q94

What's the most reliable and easy way to slim and maintain weight loss?

The two things people dread, long-term, are weighing and measuring all their food and constantly having to look things up in a calorie/fat guide. This can be boring and time-consuming and, of course, everyone is looking for an easier way to keep the weight off for good. In my experience, it's good to do these things for a week or two – actually finding out what, say, an ounce of Cheddar or a 100ml portion of ice-cream looks like is quite interesting and eye-opening. A modicum of knowledge gives your slimming and maintenance diet the greatest chance of success. Even if you follow a diet in a book, you still almost always have to weigh or measure at least some items.

The good news is that, after a while, you come to know what portion sizes look like and, broadly speaking, what foods you should be cutting back on, which to avoid and which to eat freely. This is sometimes called the 'traffic light system' (see Question 95). Eating this way should result in fairly easy – and healthy – steady slimming and long-term weight maintenance. A few simple fat-cutting tips help make the system easier.

you and your food

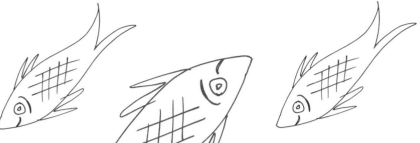

Which brings me nicely to the crux of your question. A reduced-fat, high-complex-carb (majoring on low-GI carbs, see Question 66) natural diet, low in processed and sugary foods, saturates and trans fats, and adequate in protein, is the easiest and most reliable way to get and stay slim that is also nutritionally sound and healthy. Both the World Health Organization and the US Department of Agriculture agree on this – as do most health and diet professionals.

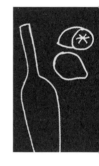

I have to admit that I know people who have got – and stayed – slim over time via other means. A high-protein, low-carb diet is, arguably, easier than low-fat, high-carb eating and also reliable, although for long-term weight maintenance, compliance (sticking with it) may not be so good. The Hay system (food combining) is favoured by many and is probably a reliable way to stay slim, though not exactly easy to follow. The Hay system is fairly healthy, while high-protein eating generally is not.

In the long-term, if you think 'healthy eating' and 'fat cutting', then you shouldn't go far wrong... oh, and 'regular exercise'. All studies show that the people most successful at keeping lost weight off are those who take regular exercise. The more calories you burn up, the more you can eat without putting on weight again!

**What is the 'traffic
light guide' to eating
for weight loss?**

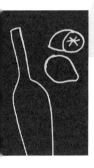

This guide to eating helps by flagging foods to cut back
on, which to avoid and which to eat freely. Eating this way
should result in easy, steady – and healthy – slimming and
long-term weight maintenance (see Question 94).

EAT FREELY: Fresh/frozen fruit and veg (except those listed elsewhere);
potatoes and other roots; salad veg; herbs and spices; wholegrains,
wholewheat pasta, wholemeal bread, wholegrain breakfast cereals; dried
apricots, prunes; all pulses; all fish and shellfish; low-fat yoghurt, low-fat
cheeses (e.g. cottage cheese), fromage frais, skimmed milk; poultry
(skinless) and game; Quorn, tofu.

EAT IN MODERATION: Refined grains (e.g. white bread); good-quality
cooking oils (e.g. olive or groundnut oil); dried fruits (except those listed
above); full-fat yoghurt, semi-skimmed milk, full-fat fromage frais;
medium-fat cheeses (e.g. Brie, Edam, goats' cheese, feta); eggs; lean red
meat; fresh nuts and seeds (not salted, roasted); processed and deli
meats; low-fat spread; fruit juices; alcohol.

AVOID, HAVE INFREQUENTLY OR IN SMALL OR VERY SMALL
QUANTITIES: Cakes, biscuits, chocolate, sweets, puddings, butter,
margarine, cream, pastry, salty snacks, full-fat cheeses, fatty meat and
meat products, sugary drinks, deep-fried foods.

you and your food

Q96

High-fat dairy products, like butter and full-fat cheeses, are high in calories and among the main sources of saturated fat. It is thus generally a good idea to cut right back on them, though they needn't be completely avoided as part of a varied diet, even when slimming. Medium- or low-fat dairy produce is better, as it is lower in fat and calories but still contains good amounts of calcium, protein, vitamins and minerals.

Giving up dairy produce altogether is unnecessary for slimming and, because it is our main source of calcium, may well be unwise unless you know enough about nutrition to get alternative sources in the right quantities, or take a supplement. Calcium is necessary for building and maintaining bones and teeth, and for a variety of other bodily functions. As with wheat, dairy produce is currently 'out of fashion', but there is no evidence that avoiding items like skimmed milk, cottage cheese, eggs and yoghurt will help a diet.

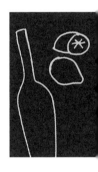

you and your food

139

Could a food allergy be causing my inability to lose weight?

A true allergy produces a very quick and often very obvious effect – e.g. a rash, vomiting, asthma. In some cases, eating a food to which you're allergic produces a life-threatening anaphylactic shock. If you have no such symptoms it's unlikely you have a genuine food allergy.

Food intolerance is the term used to describe a less severe reaction to a food, which may produce symptoms like tiredness, bowel upsets and bloating. Some people do indeed find themselves intolerant of a food or foods – with wheat, dairy and sugar being the three favourite culprits. Claims that up to 75% of the population have food intolerances are wildly exaggerated. Official estimates from the UK Food Standards Agency suggest only 2% of people may have genuine cases.

Some real food allergies can actually cause weight loss (see next question). Food intolerances often show up as stomach bloating and the foods most prone to cause this seem to be wheat (particularly wheat bran) and high-fat foods. If one of these is your problem, and you eliminate it from your diet for a week, bloating should subside and you may feel better. However, apart from the bloating effect, there is little evidence that food intolerance can actually cause weight gain. It would be impossible for a food to put more fat on you than it contains in calories – to get fat, you need to create a calorie excess. Obviously, if you give up a range of foods, as often advised by 'allergy clinics', from dairy products and wheat to sugar, alcohol, etc. you'll undoubtedly lose weight, as you'll be cutting out a lot of calories. If you're overweight and eating such items, it also follows that they may well be causing your weight problem, but it's more likely to be due to their calories than any intolerance!

Though hospital testing for allergies is reliable, currently the only reliable way to discover if you have a food intolerance is to follow an elimination diet (excluding each possible culprit food for a fortnight and noting the effect). All but the most simple elimination diets need to be done with the help of a dietitian.

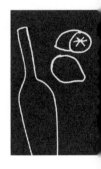

Private food allergy consultancies (testing blood, hair, nails, etc.) have, by and large, been found to be unreliable when tested by undercover researchers. Not only did they advise people to give up a range of good, healthy foods to which they aren't intolerant, but they also missed genuine allergies, which may be dangerous.

Your doctor will probably be of more help than a private clinic – she/he can refer you to a dietitian or even an allergy specialist. Lastly, it is common for people with eating disorders to seek to be diagnosed as allergic to, or intolerant of, foods like wheat and dairy as a legitimate way to avoid them.

Q98 **Does avoiding wheat products help you lose weight?**

Since several celebrities lost weight on a wheat-free diet, some people believe this is THE only way to lose weight. As a read through this chapter shows, there is little magic about a wheat-free diet for most of us. However, if you have been eating a lot of wheat (say, bread for breakfast, sandwiches for lunch and pasta for your evening meal) and then you cut it out, you will almost certainly lose weight, because you are reducing your total calorie intake. You will also find any problems with fluid retention minimized, because wheat and starchy carbs tend to retain more fluid in the body than a diet low in carbohydrates. Many people also report that on a wheat-free diet they feel better – more alert, less sluggish. There is, however, little scientific evidence that I can find to support this, except that high-carb foods tend to be 'comforters'.

Many people avoid wheat because they say they are allergic to or intolerant of it. Read the answer to the previous question and come back to this. It may be that our bodies aren't designed to cope with large amounts of wheat and for some people simply getting a variety of other foods and sources of starch in the diet is enough to avoid bloating and other possible symptoms of intolerance. You won't be missing many vital nutrients by giving up items high in refined white flour, which usually often contain other not-so-goodies, like sugar and fat. Indeed, new research shows that a diet high in highly-refined carbs, such as white bread and white flour (and other high-GI carbs, see Question 66), does encourage the body to store fat, especially around the midriff. However, wholegrain wheat is a good source of dietary fibre, complex carbohydrates, vitamins and minerals, and shouldn't be abandoned on a whim.

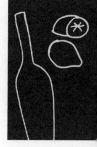

You can do a one- or two-week wheat elimination and see if you lose weight and feel better afterwards. Be warned, though, wheat is contained in very many products, including lots of commercial items on the supermarket shelves, so you will need to become an avid label-reader. If you simply replace wheat with a similar amount of other starches, such as potatoes or rice, I doubt whether you will lose much weight, but you may like to try just to satisfy yourself.

Lastly, genuine gluten allergy – an allergy to the gluten in wheat, rye, barley and oats – produces the condition called coeliac disease, one of the symptoms of which may be weight loss, along with a variety of other symptoms, such as anaemia, lethargy and painful joints. This needs to be treated professionally.

Q99

Are there disadvantages to diets restricted to just a few types of food?

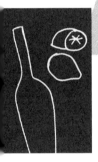

You may suffer from nutritional deficiencies on the one hand, and a surfeit of other nutrients on the other. For example, on a diet of only carrots and apples, you'd get too much beta-carotene (which can turn skin yellow and poison you) and little protein, essential fats and a range of vitamins and minerals.

The second disadvantage is that you'll probably get extremely bored with the same few foods and more likely to give up – though, in the short term, people seem to tolerate reduced-choice diets well. This is because they take away the worry and indecision. However, these reasons aren't enough to recommend such a diet.

The third disadvantage is that, in the long term, any weight lost on such a diet is unlikely to stay off, as you haven't learnt more sensible eating habits.

A fourth reason is that it is the overall calorie deficit created that matters, not what foods you eat or avoid. Whether you eat, say, 1,500 calories a day on a varied diet or 1,500 calories of apples and carrots, weight loss will be much the same.

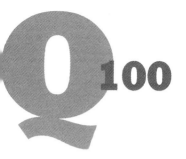

Q100

I enjoy fast food, like burgers and chips. Is it really necessary to cut these out to lose weight and keep it off?

Most fast food is surprisingly high in fat. So, from both dieting and health viewpoints, a regular diet of it isn't a great idea. Even items you might think aren't high in fat, like chicken or vegetarian burgers, coleslaw or a salad main meal, usually are (see Question 101). For example, a McDonald's Vegetable Deluxe contains nearly 19g of fat – over double that in their hamburger!

Of course, you can have the occasional treat even on a slimming diet – nearly all food has at least some good points: for example, a beefburger is high in iron and protein, B vitamins and zinc (the bun's OK too – the fat's in the fries and mayo.) Some takeouts ARE much lower in fat than others – such as lower-fat, all-vegetable pizza and tandoori chicken.

Another idea is to prepare 'takeaway'-type meals at home, where you can control content (Question 106). However, some takeaway addicts turn up their noses at 'healthier' options, which just don't do it for them. A read of the You and Your Health and Fitness chapter may provide motivation on the health score.

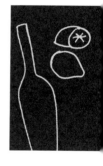

you and your food

145

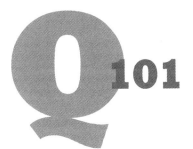

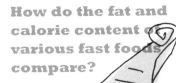

Q101

How do the fat and calorie content of various fast foods compare?

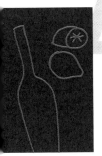

The following are approximate contents of average portions of some popular fast foods:

Fried cod/chips 1,000 cals 55g fat;
Large doner kebab/pitta 700 cals 40g fat

CHINESE Chicken chow mein 700 cals 14g fat; Peking duck 750 cals 25g fat
Sweet-and-sour pork 500 cals 18g fat Crispy pancake roll (1) 240 cals 10g fat

INDIAN Beef Madras 550 cals 20g fat; Chicken tikka masala 680 cals 40g fat
Tandoori chicken 320 cals 8g fat; Onion bhaji (1) 190 cals 16g fat

THAI Red beef curry 650 cals 20g fat; Green chicken curry 600 cals 18g fat

PIZZA (whole individual pizza) Spicy meat 850 cals 42g fat
Margherita 650 cals 23g fat; Marinara 525 cals 13g fat
Pepperoni 800 cals 14g fat

BURGERS/CHICKEN Quarterpounder/cheese/reg fries 750 cals 37g fat
Quarterpounder in bun 425 cals 20g fat
Chicken fillet burger/reg fries 700 cals 32g fat
Chicken nuggets (6 pieces) 250 cals 15g fat; 2 drumsticks 370 cals 22g fat

TEX-MEX Beef enchiladas 650 cals 30g fat; Chicken fajitas 725 cals 30g fat
Nachos 450 cals 20g fat

Q102

I love chocolate – can I eat is as part of a slimming diet?

Yes, but not in the same quantities. You could fit a daily 250-calorie bar into a 1,500 calories/day diet, but not on the type of diet that seems to work best – about 25% fat content. 50g milk chocolate contains about 250 calories and 15g fat, 9g saturated, over a third of daily fat intake and more than the whole saturates intake. So, on a low-fat diet, only about 100 calories a day of chocolate fit in.

Instead, find ways to get the taste with fewer calories (below), or designate one day a week as 'chocolate day' and allow yourself your favourite bar then. This only works if you're not a 'chocoholic' (see Question 123). Chocolate cravings can be due to low blood sugar (Questions 63-8).

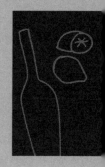

Chocolate taste for less

• Low-calorie hot chocolate drinks – about 40 calories.
• Strawberries dipped into melted chocolate – 15 calories per strawberry.
• Small amount of good-quality dark chocolate – more satisfying than a larger amount of cheaper chocolate and good for your heart because of its antioxidants. Two squares – about 50 calories.

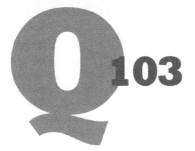

Q103

I have a sweet tooth and can't live without desserts – any suggestions?

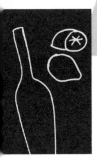

The solution is to base desserts around fruit, which is naturally sweet but not high in calories – and also good for you. If fresh fruit is not 'desserty' enough for you, try:

• Baked bananas (bake in their skins until black and serve with a sprinkling of brown sugar and lemon juice) – about 100 calories a portion.

• Summer puddings made in the usual way but with half the quantity of fructose instead of sugar – about 200 calories per 125g (5oz) slice, served with Greek yoghurt (15ml, 16 cals per tbsp).

• Fruit kebabs, brushed with low-fat spread and grilled or barbecued – about 50 calories per stick.

• Fruit fools made by whizzing rhubarb, gooseberries or strawberries with a little fructose and 0%-fat fromage frais – about 125 calories per 150ml ($^1/_4$ pint).

• Fruit layers made with puréed or whole soft fruits and Greek yoghurt, topped with no-added-sugar muesli – about 150 calories per 150ml ($^1/_4$ pint) portion.

Desserts based on fruit and calcium-rich dairy produce are not items to feel guilty about, so you win all ways.

Q104

I adore cheese (all the full-fat kinds) – how can my diet cope with its calories?

Like the chocolate lover in Question 102, you need to find ways to get the flavour without the calories:
• Buy best-quality, strong cheeses, such as mature farmhouse Cheddar or Parmesan – much smaller quantities satisfy the taste buds.
• Grate cheese for sandwiches; you use much less.
• Mix grated cheese with grated carrot for a salad; again it goes further.
• Make a low-cal sauce with sauce flour, skimmed milk and a little grated strong cheese for pasta, fish and fish pies.
• Blue cheeses tend to be tangier, so you need less. Some are lower in calories than others – e.g. Danish Blue or Irish Cashel Blue.
• Both feta and most medium-mature goats' cheeses are medium-fat, high in taste and tang, and can therefore be used in small quantities – both are good in salads.
Small amounts of most cheeses can be included in any slimming diet – even a low-fat one. Cheese is high in calcium and protein. Cheese addiction may, in fact, be salt addiction – most cheese is very high in salt.

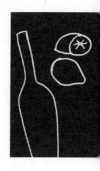

Q105

What are the best (quick and/or easy) cooking methods for slimmers?

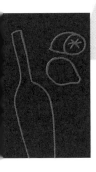

Well, there's plenty of scope. The only method that is probably unwise for slimmers is deep-frying. An easy cooking method is tray-baking, perhaps with a little olive oil. This can be used for almost all vegetables, meat and fish. Stir-frying is simple and, if you eat meat, fish and poultry, marinating lean cuts and then grilling or barbecuing takes a lot of beating for flavour and ease. If I were vegetarian, I would virtually live on salads, stews and soups!

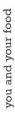

Q106

What are the best tips for reducing calories in my food painlessly?

Some tips for reducing calories painlessly:
- Use cooking oil spray to coat non-stick frying pans.
- When a stir-fry goes dry, add a little water, not more fat.
- Use 8%-fat fromage frais or smetana in desserts, dips and sauces instead of full-fat yoghurt or cream.
- Reduce portions by 20%, except veg and salad – increase them 50%.
- Let casseroles and stews go cold and remove any fat that rises to the surface, before reheating and serving.
- Make fat-free béchamel with sauce flour and skim milk.

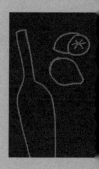

Homemade takeaways
- Extra-lean quarterpounder with potato wedges coated in herb seasoning before baking, salad (about 400 cals).
- Chicken pieces (skinless) coated in yoghurt and Mexican herb mixture, baked and served with baked potato skins and home-made guacamole – mashed avocado, tomato, chilli and spring onion (about 450 cals).
- Pitta pizza – top a pitta with tomato sauce, grated mozzarella cheese and slices of tomato, red onion and yellow pepper and grill until bubbling (about 350 cals).

you and your food

151

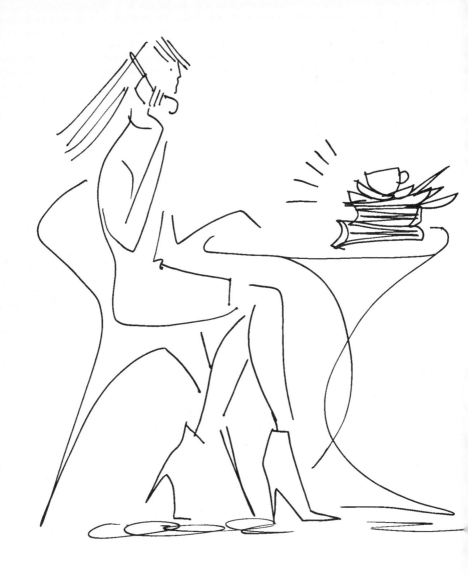

For many, the psychological, emotional and practical problems of eating to get – and stay – slim seem almost insurmountable. Ever since gluttony was named as one of the seven deadly sins, the inhabitants of the Western world have had to contend with feelings of guilt about eating. It is this dichotomy – knowing that food is something we want, crave, need, but is also something we can so easily come to fear or even hate – that we need to resolve.

In this section, we aim to unravel the mystery – and, often, misery – of our relationship with food. You want to stay slim; you want to lose weight – but healthy, non-fattening food just doesn't seem to fit in with your lifestyle. Many of us are too busy and stressed to want to pay attention to diet or cooking. We work hard and play hard – yet when it comes to food, we are ambivalent. We buy cookery books to adorn our kitchens but – statistics show – rarely sit down to a proper family meal any more. In this section I hope to help unravel some of these strands with coherent solutions.

you and your life

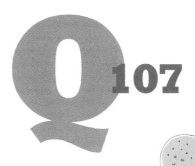

Q107

I know I should lose
weight – but how do
I get motivated?

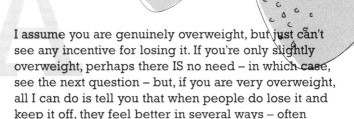

I assume you are genuinely overweight, but just can't
see any incentive for losing it. If you're only slightly
overweight, perhaps there IS no need – in which case,
see the next question – but, if you are very overweight,
all I can do is tell you that when people do lose it and
keep it off, they feel better in several ways – often
unexpected ones.

In 1997 the *American Journal of Clinical Nutrition*
published a review of how people felt after they'd lost
weight. The slimmers said the quality of their lives had
improved in the following ways: general quality of life
(95%); level of energy (92%); mobility (92%); general
mood (91%); self-confidence (91%); physical health
(86%); interactions with strangers (69%); interactions
with opposite sex (65%); interactions with spouse
(56%); job performance (54%); hobbies (49%). By the
way, I take the quaint expression 'interactions' to mean
people agreeing to come on a date with you, or your
spouse allowing you back into the matrimonial bed.
These findings match those from my own observations

of the many people I've helped to slim over the years. People blossom after losing weight!

It might be useful for you to write a list of all the ways you think you'd feel if you were slim. Also write a list of the health benefits you think you want. You could also attempt to add up all the lost days or hours you have spent fretting about not being more slim, or feeling guilty about eating too much. For most people that comes to a large chunk of their adult lives.

You must decide – do I accept my weight and live happily with it, or do I really want to change? The worst motivation for slimming is saying, 'I should...', 'I must...', 'I'd better...' or 'My doctor says...' If you aren't doing it because you want to and believe that you can, then it's not likely that you will succeed.

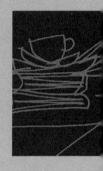

One trick if you want to but aren't sure that you can – i.e., you're halfway there – is to think yourself into the part. This idea – called by American actor Roy Scheider 'Acting Well' – uses techniques advocated by Stanislavski's method school of acting. You create your thin self in your mind and think about what you do, how you look, what you eat, what exercise you do, how popular you are. Over time, you become what you are imagining in a natural way. You eat better, take more exercise, lose weight, and turn into your 'thin self'. It worked for Roy, and he also used the same method to give up smoking.

Another tool is to join a slimming club – the comradeship and common goal works for many. Getting weighed every week is also a great motivator!

Q108

I've lost weight before and it all returns – what's the point?

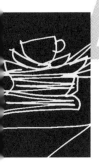

Research reveals a third of slimmers gain up to an extra stone after each successive dieting period, also that constant fluctuating weight can damage the immune system and people who stay slightly overweight may be healthier long term than yo-yo dieters.

If your BMI is no more than 25–7, you may be better off simply trying not to put on more weight. Aiming too low is an important factor in yo-yoing, so if you do try again, set a realistic target. Also, don't set out to 'diet', but to eat better, and to look at your whole lifestyle. Do you take exercise? Are you stressed? What causes you to overeat? Joining a group like Overeaters Anonymous might be good.

Weight loss for previous dieters is better when a side effect of something fun. My neighbour was plump until she and her husband got into line-dancing, ending up with them out dancing 5 nights a week. Within a year she'd shed 3 stones. She's fit, happy and eats what she wants.

The point is getting the maintenance right, not just the slimming. There IS no point to dieting, unless you have a long-term strategy, ideally including regular exercise.

you and your life

156

Q109

Everyone tells me diets don't work – so why bother?

First read the two previous questions, which may help to resolve the 'why bother' point. Now, on to the first part of your question. Diets DO work. If you eat fewer calories than your body uses, you'll lose weight.

What people mean by 'diets don't work' is that the weight tends to return... and then some. This IS true – in most studies, about 95% of people have put back all their weight after a year. Other studies, however, show that certain people – notably those who begin to take regular exercise – DO keep the weight off.

From my own experience, it's those who run, cycle, walk, swim, dance, enjoy the outdoors, garden, have active jobs and so on who seem most successful in keeping their youthful figures into middle age. It doesn't take a lot. Burning just 100 extra calories a day in, say, a half-hour walk, could mean that you save yourself from putting on a whole stone in weight over a year.

So diets DO work – but you need to commit yourself to a regular activity programme to keep the weight off.

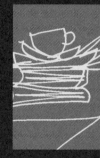

you and your life

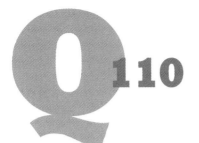

Q110

Everyone tells me I look just fine as I am – so why should I slim?

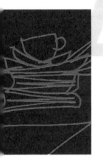

Perhaps you do look fine, and perhaps you shouldn't slim. Read Question 26 to find out. If it shows you do need to lose weight on health grounds, then I would trust this rather than what people say. Well-meaning friends will almost always say, 'Oh, you look fine!' especially in response to a heartfelt query from you along the lines of, 'Do you think I'm too fat?'

However, all research shows that we live in a fat-prejudiced society. The World Health Organization reports that obesity is 'highly stigmatized in industrialized countries', even down to doctors being less interested in treating obese patients. The Association for the Study of Obesity says that very fat students are 65% less likely to get a place at college, even if they have the same grades; that they are less likely to get a job or promotion, and that, in Britain, obese women are paid on average 5% less.

Unfair though all this is, it is a fact at the moment. Choose whether or not to lose weight with unbiased advice – friends are the last people to ask.

Q111

I'd like to lose weight but my family don't want me to - what do I do?

It's strange how we don't like our own fat bodies, but if our nearest and dearest are fat and want to lose weight we panic! Families like familiarity, and they know and love you as you are now. However, there could also be a less altruistic motive. People who lose weight can change quite drastically – becoming more confident, more selfish even. The family may realize this (albeit subconsciously) and want to keep you 'in line'. They see your losing weight as a threat. An under-confident spouse may wonder if you'll be swept off your feet by a newer model when slim again.

So, this is more common than you might think. What to do? Quietly get on with slimming and carry on other areas of life as normal. If you do it slowly and sensibly, and don't make a big issue of it, all should be fine. If you do feel much better when slim (which you will) and make life changes, then you and the family can deal with them when they happen. Don't stay fat because your family want you to.

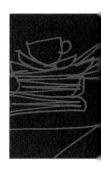

We live in a food-
dominated society –
how can I slim when
the odds seem
stacked against me?

I think this is THE big and crucial question. Indeed, it
does seem as though the odds are stacked against
individuals trying to lose weight, when all around is a
non-stop, relentless onslaught of food promotion. Media
advertising, supermarket specials, fast food, street food,
dining out, eating with friends, snack food sold almost
everywhere from DIY stores to newsagents. Everything
is geared to try to persuade us to eat and drink more
than we need or want.

Over-production of food is the biggest cause of
obesity in the USA. The nation produces nearly 4,000
calories of food a day for every citizen (including
children) – double the average calorie requirement. The
food industry is the biggest industry in the world. Never
let anyone try to kid you that it is the diet industry that
makes billions off our fat backs; it is the food producers
and retailers who do that. We get fat – and then what
happens? We are the ones who end up feeling
inadequate and guilty, greedy and weak-willed.

It is NOT all your fault you are fat. However, I still do

think that it IS up to the individual – having recognized that people are trying to get rich on your liking for fatty foods, sugary foods, salty foods, snacks, alcohol, or just too much of everything – to put up resistance. Try to recognize the ploys used every day to get you to eat or drink when you don't need to eat or drink, and get in the habit of tuning in to your own real hunger signals and food and nutrition needs rather than listening to these 'devils in disguise'.

It may take a while, but you can retrain your taste buds to enjoy more natural, less fattening, healthier foods, and you can train your appetite to let you know what they're really thinking. This way you end up eating when YOU want or need to eat, what YOU want or need to eat, and in quantities that YOU decide are right. It doesn't take willpower, but determination.

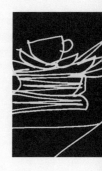

You could also read up on the way mass-market food is produced – John Humphrys' book *The Great Food Gamble* (Hodder, £12.99) is an eye-opener. If you thought you enjoyed fast food, and all kinds of other consumer foods, you may change your mind after you read this and decide that it's organic for you from now on! You could also become a campaigner yourself – things won't change unless enough people demand better-quality food, and stricter advertising standards, and that the food giants – and the government – don't hinder, but help us to help ourselves in the war of the weight.

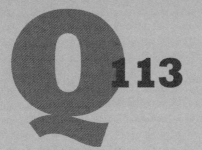

Q113

Food is my main pleasure – why should I deny myself?

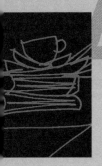

Many people who live to eat do get fat, but having food as a main pleasure doesn't necessarily dispose you to fatness. Food is one of my real pleasures, but over a few years I've come to enjoy different eating patterns and foods. Why the change? See the previous question – and I've learnt to regard my body as important and want to feed it well – not the same as overindulging it. 'Indulgence' to me now means feasting on tasty natural foods.

There is also, of course, a difference between having food as your 'main pleasure' and as 'a pleasure'. Try the following, which may help you make small changes that add up to a big difference:

• Follow the retraining framework in Question 133.
• Replace rich, fatty, salty or sugary foods with other strong tastes and aromatic foods that are less fattening.
• Listen to your body and begin reading signals. Are you really hungry? Are you full? Act on them.
• Always eat slowly and chew thoroughly – you may naturally eat less.
• Don't deny yourself good food, but rethink parameters.

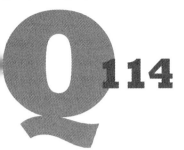

Q114

Isn't it true that overweight people are just basically greedy and lazy?

A WHO report on obesity says it's clear that it's not simply a result of overindulgence or lack of physical activity. Although anyone can create an energy deficit and lose weight, some people are much more predisposed to putting on weight.

Generally weight gain happens gradually (mostly between 25 and 50), and it doesn't take much overeating to gain even a stone. If you eat just one large slice of bread and butter a day more than you need (about 150 calories), in a year you'd put on about 15lb (7kg). Moreover, temptation is all around us – it's more a matter of food always being there so we eat it, rather than greed.

It's also true that most of us don't take enough exercise – the Government says we use on average 800 calories a day less in activity than we did in 1970. Exercise is by far the best way to prevent long-term weight gain – but it would be unfair to describe people who don't take enough exercise as 'lazy'. Mostly people have got out of the habit of fitting exercise into their hectic lives.

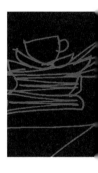

you and your life

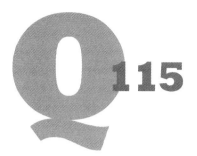

Q 115

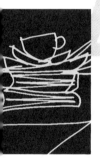

There's really no such thing as 'diet' food. A good slimmer's diet can be filled with great tastes and textures, colours and aromas. The days of 'cottage cheese, cardboard crispbread and limp lettuce' are thankfully long gone.

New research indicates that overweight people hate bland diets because they have a greater need for strong flavours. So they don't try slimming diets because they perceive them to be boring and bland. However, calorie- and fat-reduced diets have become much more sophisticated, as we now know exactly how to cut unnecessary calories while retaining loads of interest, flavour and satisfaction – as well as a decent-sized plateful.

I think the way to ensure food is kept exciting and enticing, is to go big on ethnic eating... the spices of the Middle East and India, the herbs and vegetables of the Mediterranean, the more exotic grains and pulses. What could be better than chicken spiced with coriander, cumin and chilli, or a delicious Greek salad with feta, or a plate of pasta sprinkled with fresh basil and balsamic vinegar? All these are, or can be, staples of a calorie-reduced diet.

you and your life

164

Q116

What are the best tips for delicious dieting?

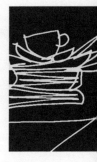

• Pulse and meat casseroles (beef and kidney beans, lean lamb and chickpeas). Brown meat in non-stick pan sprayed with low-cal cooking spray. Use good stock, herbs, passata.
• Vegetable curries: mix root and other veg/pulses and use fresh spices for maximum flavour. Use ½ tablespoon vegetable oil per person for frying onion and spices. Good combinations include: potato and spinach, aubergine and lentils. Thicken with yoghurt. Use chilli, ginger, cumin, coriander seeds and leaves, good vegetable stock.
• Ethnic salads: combine robust salad leaves with fruity/spicy low-fat dressings and add low-fat protein (e.g. chicken, turkey, fish) plus one or two other veg and/or fruits and some starch (e.g. pasta, potatoes, rice). Good combinations are fresh tuna with tomatoes and courgettes, bulgar wheat with goats' cheese. Use fresh salad herbs, good vinegar or citrus juice, extra-virgin olive oil.

Foods that add flavour for few calories: Vegetables: red peppers, mushrooms, rocket; Fish: tuna, salmon, monkfish; Spices: cumin, fennel, ginger; Herbs: basil, mint, tarragon; Flavourings: balsamic vinegar, soy sauce, mustard.

you and your life

165

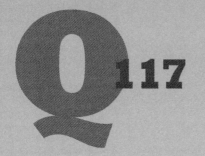

Q117

Can you recommend a strategy to beat comfort eating on carbohydrates?

Eating carbohydrate foods for comfort may have some basis in physical need. For example, eating foods very high in sugars and starches and low in protein may increase the activity of the neurotransmitter serotonin in the brain, involved in the control of mood and behaviour (the drug Prozac works by promoting serotonin activity). So, in effect, you may be 'dosing' yourself with carbs to try to treat depression. There is circumstantial evidence for this in that people who suffer from seasonal affective disorder (SAD), who get depressed in the winter, automatically increase carb intake at that time.

Another possible cause may be that you aren't eating regularly enough and a sudden urge for carbs may be due to low blood sugar. The British Nutrition Foundation reported in 2001 that dieters are more likely to turn to food for comfort when under stress than other people, and this may be linked to blood sugar – or simply because dieters can be 'good' when not stressed, but if things go wrong, it may be 'blow the diet' – yet another reason to avoid strict very-low-calorie diets and to slim slowly.

The consensus is that the likely reasons for eating carbs when miserable are simply that they are pleasurable to eat and temporarily help ease negative feelings. Some people turn to alcohol, shopping, etc. while others turn to food if they have problems. If you feel you're actually depressed, you should visit your doctor, who may recommend medication and/or refer you for counselling.

If you just eat for comfort when feeling 'fed up', the following strategies may help:

• Eat small regular meals, so when you feel below par you may be slightly less inclined to overeat. Don't ever be over-strict on yourself about food.

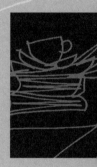

• Prepare ahead alternative 'comforters' – if you know you regularly eat chocolate, say, in a crisis, think of alternative things that may help you feel better, say, soothing music.

• Distract yourself when you feel the urge for carbs coming on. If hungry, eat something other than carbs (e.g. a little cheese). Get away from the kitchen and do something else – have a bath or go for a walk.

• Remember, just because you have a craving, it doesn't mean you have to do anything about it. Keep telling yourself you're in control and eventually you will be.

• Reflect on what's causing you to comfort eat and see what can be done to alter or improve the situation. This is the most important part of the strategy in the long term. If food is filling a hole in your emotional life, or acting as a support system or a mask for problems, then you may not find it easy to control until you sort out the underlying reasons. You may also like to join a group like Overeaters Anonymous.

you and your life

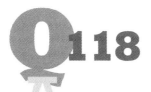

Q118

How do I stop eating when bored, evenings and weekends?

A survey reveals that almost half of adults eat through boredom or loneliness. Sounds as if you have an enjoyable job but haven't done enough to ensure balance in your life. You need to spend time thinking about yourself, your aims, your interests. The answer to loneliness is involvement with others – but how? What would you enjoy? As to lack of purpose, you need things that'll make you feel useful. Whatever the reasons for your boredom and consequent overeating, you need to tackle both long-term with lifestyle changes.

Q119

I eat when I'm angry and/or frustrated – is there a cure?

Some smoke, others drink or take drugs, you eat. Eating to suppress anger has been described as, literally, pushing the anger back down inside yourself with the food. You need to address the causes of your anger, if it's frequent, and see what you can do to minimize or rid yourself of them. If you can't do this on your own, you'd probably benefit from counselling or sessions with a group like Overeaters Anonymous.

you and your life

168

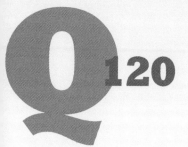

Q 120

I've got no willpower at all, so I can never stick to a diet – any tips?

I don't like the word 'willpower' because, if huge efforts of will are needed non-stop during a slimming campaign, then I believe it's bound to fail. I prefer 'determination', for certainly you need to be determined and motivated in order to lose weight.

So first examine your own motivations (see Question 107) and come up with the main reasons you want to slim. Next you need to set a sensible target weight, so you aren't trying to diet too low. Now pick a suitable food intake level so that you aren't permanently hungry – Question 85 will help here. Then you need to make sensible food choices, which will also help you to feel sated and happy while you slim.

You may find the support of a slimming club helpful to you – many people find the better ones extremely motivating. You may also benefit from trying the retraining framework in Question 133. You will definitely benefit from regular exercise. The more you do, the more you can eat and still lose weight.

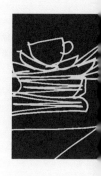

you and your life

169

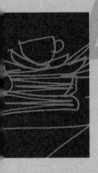

Many people have forgotten how it feels to be truly hungry – regular mealtimes and snacks mean our stomachs are rarely empty long enough to register hunger. We eat because it's time to eat. So your need for food may well be more habit than hunger, and if we all just ate when we were genuinely hungry, we wouldn't be fat.

How to tell the difference? It's interesting to keep a food diary and record what you ate, when and why. In the 'why' column, you'll find reasons, like, 'Had a pizza while Sue and I went shopping – because we always do.' Not all your reasons will come down to habit, but many will.

We're creatures of habit, we love our rituals, and food and drink fit neatly into them. The cure? A good first step is to become aware of what you're doing (keep that food diary going in your head) and before you eat ask yourself, 'Is it hunger or habit?' Begin saying 'no' to the food, at least some of the time. Eventually it gets easier, because you get more in tune with your real hunger signals.

Q122

What's the difference between greed and hunger?

It's said that when you eat food because you fancy it, that's greed, and when you eat because you need to, that's hunger. However, this is an over-simplification. Hunger comes after a reasonable period without food and may be enhanced by fresh air and exercise. If you can match one of these criteria and have a 'grumbling' tummy, then you're probably hungry.

Greed isn't a word I like – 'over-enthusiastic appetite' may be better. Even if you're not hungry, appetite can be triggered by the appearance of a 'novel' food (one you haven't just eaten, say dessert after a large meal) or by a favourite food. Between-meal snacks may also be eaten because of the 'moreish' factor, not hunger. Snack foods like chocolate aren't regarded as 'staple' foods and tend to be used as treats or rewards. However, they may also be eaten when you're genuinely hungry (not a good idea, see Question 67).

When not genuinely hungry you're unlikely to choose, say, a salad – but an item high in fat and/or sugar and/or refined starch. If hungry, you'll eat anything.

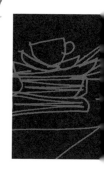

you and your life

171

Q123

I'm a chocoholic. Can chocolate be addictive, like drugs?

Chocolate isn't addictive in the sense drugs can be, but its key ingredient, the cocoa bean, does contain chemicals blamed for causing addiction – the methylxanthines, a group of stimulants, including caffeine, theobromine and theophylline. It also contains phenylethylamine (PEA), which can cause migraine in some, but also has properties similar to amphetamine, and can enhance levels of natural painkiller endorphins. It's also said to increase libido and is the same chemical as that produced in the bodies of people in love. Cocoa beans are also said to contain a cannabis-like relaxant, amandamide.

However, it seems chocolate itself usually doesn't contain enough of these chemicals to produce 'addiction' (white chocolate contains hardly any). The British Nutrition Foundation recently concluded levels of methylxanthines in chocolate are so small they are unlikely to have any effect, and that the phenylethylamine in it cannot influence mood. 40g of milk chocolate provides only 10mg caffeine – a tiny percentage of that in a cup of strong coffee – and dark chocolate has about half that of a cup of tea.

you and your life

172

The other oft-cited effect of chocolate is that, as it's a high-carbohydrate food (high in sugar), it increases brain serotonin (see Question 117) and therefore makes us feel happy. In fact, the BNF reports, foods containing more than very small amounts of protein – as chocolate does in its milk and/or cocoa content – don't have this effect.

The answer, then, to why chocolate is so moreish is that a) it melts at blood temperature, providing a uniquely pleasurable sensation in the mouth, b) it does release the body's natural endorphins simply because of the pleasure, and c) it provides a hedonistic buzz because it's 'naughty'.

Is there a cure for a chocolate 'addiction'? You may benefit from the retraining in Question 133. A good trick is to have chocolate as part of something substantial, say a chocolate-coated muesli bar, as normally chocolate slips down so quickly you eat too much before you think you've had enough. Researchers found that smelling vanilla blunts appetite for chocolate – so try vanilla candles or essence. It's also important to keep blood-sugar levels even to prevent cravings (see Question 127).

There's good news though. In moderation, chocolate is good for health, containing antioxidant polyphenols that can help protect against heart disease. The University of California reported that 40g of dark chocolate contains double the antioxidants of red wine, and several studies have confirmed its health-enhancing properties. However, milk chocolate contains less and white chocolate none.

So a little very good dark chocolate can be part of an overall healthy diet, even if slimming, and may be good for your body – and mind, as long as you never feel guilty.

Q124

I'm disorganized and hate planning – what's the best way to reduce food intake?

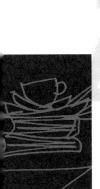

You could try the 'traffic light' system in Question 95. This is about as relaxed and informal as slimming can get – but it isn't as scientific as, say, calorie or fat counting, so weight loss, while probable, isn't 100% guaranteed.

You could simply try portion control – give yourself half-portions of your normal food and add extra portions of vegetables, salad and fruit; this works for many people and involves hardly any planning.

However, it's a pity that you don't want to give any time or thought to your diet. If you're overweight, which I assume you are, it is probably this 'mindless' eating that has made you fat. Why not consider putting your body first for a change and feed it more thoughtfully? This chapter is full of ideas for helping you eat better without too much fuss or change of lifestyle.

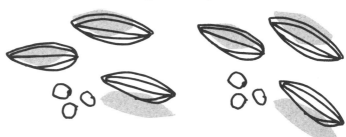

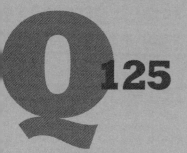

Q125

All my life I've existed on a diet of mostly junk food. How can I slim?

You should make changes gradually (see Question 133), concentrating on foods and meals that you CAN have and that you DO like, rather than fretting about what you CAN'T have and DON'T like. Even the most die-hard junk-food fan can find foods that he/she likes which are healthy and non-fattening as part of a varied diet.

Here are a few of the foods you can include on a slimming and maintenance diet without any trouble: bread, potatoes, pasta, rice, noodles, baked beans, breakfast cereals, strawberries, bananas, steak, chicken, lamb, curries, burgers and other takeaways/fast food. These are just some of the foods some people think they can't eat when slimming, but they're all good foods that contribute to a healthy slimming diet.

You'll find more help and ideas for eating elsewhere in the book. Hopefully you will gradually realize, as many people before you have, that there's plenty of enjoyment in food to be had even when you're losing weight, and that you don't have to abandon the familiar. Slimming isn't all lentils and crispbreads.

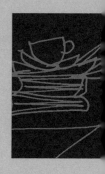

you and your life

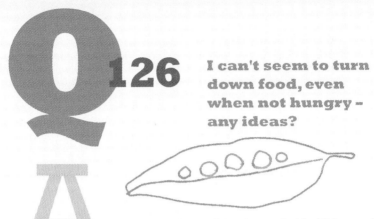

Q126

I can't seem to turn down food, even when not hungry – any ideas?

Hunger isn't your problem – false 'appetite' is. This need for food is discussed in Questions 121 and 122. I believe that you can only cure this urge – which is, basically, habit – to take what's on offer by strongly motivating yourself to say 'no', until finally saying 'no' becomes more of a habit than saying 'yes'.

I devised a system for one of my earlier books (*Slim for Life*) called 'Focus – Decide – Say No'.

• First learn to focus on what's happening. You're about to grab a biscuit on the way past the biscuit barrel, so now STOP and focus. Talk your way through the moment (under your breath may be best if anyone's about). 'Now why am I heading to grab that biscuit? Am I hungry? Do I need it? Who put that biscuit tin there?' In other words, make your brain aware of the potential calorie disaster presented to you.

• Now decide what to do and give yourself a valid reason. 'I don't want a biscuit. I'm not hungry and I know it contains 80 calories. If I have one, I'll have two or three. Then I'll feel bad. And it's only half an hour until lunch anyway.'

• Say no. Tell yourself loudly and forcibly – 'NO. I am not going to have a biscuit now.' And move away from the situation; distract yourself with something else.

To that – which you do every time you are about to eat something you're not hungry for – I'd add a fourth element.

• Look at ways to stop yourself even being in that situation. To prevent the biscuit incident, literally move the biscuit barrel into a cupboard where it is out of sight and mind or, even better, ditch the biscuit barrel altogether and stop buying biscuits.

There are always ways round 'temptation incidents'. For example, if you are going round to a friend's house for coffee, ask him/her beforehand please not to put out any cake. End of problem. Think of your most frequent temptation times and see if you can think of strategies to defuse them now, so that you don't even have to 'Focus – Decide – Say No'.

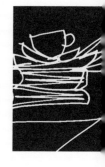

In the long term, realize that we aren't living in times of famine and that you don't have to 'stock up' calorie supplies in case you don't get anything to eat for ages. Researchers in the US say that obese Americans (a large percentage of their population) panic unless they are within sight of a food source because of this ancient urge to eat while the going's good.

Q127

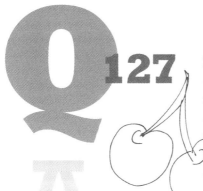

I can easily go all day with virtually no food, but in the evening, especially in winter, I crave food – mostly sweet snacks. What am I doing wrong?

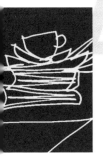

You're starving your body all day, causing low blood sugar and cravings for food that'll quickly raise blood sugar. In winter you may also suffer from seasonal affective disorder, a form of depression that can be alleviated by starchy/ sweet foods to increase mood-enhancing serotonin.

The trouble is, if you binge on sweet food on an empty stomach, insulin is released in quantity to deal with the sugar, causing blood sugar to dip too low again – so you eat more sugary foods, and so on. Here's what to do:

• Eat regularly during the day – small low-sugar healthy meals, including high-GI foods (see Question 66).

• Have your evening meal fairly early and have some nibbles by your side – try crudités – to keep you going while you prepare the meal.

• When you do have something sweet, eat it as part of a meal and not on its own.

There's no point in trying to diet by avoiding food all day. For most, it's one of the worst ways. If your cravings aren't curbed by the plan above, read Question 103 for safer ways to satisfy sweet cravings.

Q128

Is there an organization like Alcoholics Anonymous for the overweight?

The best-known one is Overeaters Anonymous, which is the ultimate self-help organization for food addicts, and has branches all over the country. They say, 'Our primary purpose is to abstain from compulsive overeating and carry the message of recovery to those who still suffer.' Telephone 07000 784985 for more information. Designated websites and chatrooms on the Internet also offer a similar type of service.

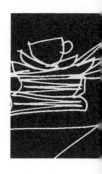

you and your life

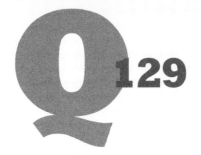

Q129

I'm overweight, but a feminist – and it's well documented that dieting is a form of female submission, isn't it?

Ever since the publication of *Fat is a Feminist Issue* there have been authors and journalists who have decried the idea that women have to be slim, and have put forward all kinds of theories as to why being slim – or trying to lose weight – is against feminist principles. Typical protests are: 'Why should we fit into an ideal that men want us to look like?'... 'Thinness is weakness, not strength – so we can be dominated.'

However, I believe that most feminists would say that their mantra is that women should make their own decisions and be true to themselves; they should be able and willing to look after themselves and to put themselves first or at least equal-first. I am also quite sure that any sensible feminist would agree that the body – male or female – is a precious tool to be looked after well, because without a strong, fit, healthy body you have lost half your natural assets, and maintaining your body at a reasonable weight is, I would have thought, one of the major self-help ways to stay healthy. Therefore, I believe that sensible concern with your size concurs with the

you and your life

feminist beliefs, rather than conflicting with them.

A read of many of the questions in this book will show you all the links that overweight and obesity have with ill health. If you're genuinely overweight, then anyone who discourages you from losing the stones on the grounds of political correctness is giving potentially dangerous advice and should, I think, be ignored.

There is no political mileage or personal happiness to be gained by staying fat if you'd rather be slimmer. However, any weight problem needs to be tackled in a sensible way. 'Diets' and 'dieting' have understandably developed a bad name over the past decade or two because of the number of people (mostly women) who diet to stick-thinness, who 'yo-yo diet', and who spend their lives ruled by food or dominated by their own need to control food. Indeed, argue feminists understandably, why replace one set of chains with another?

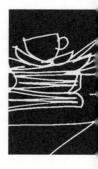

Your answer is to lose weight with a combination of moderate calorie reduction (perhaps a reduced-fat, high-complex-carb diet would suit you), coupled with an exercise regime to strengthen your muscles and get you fit, until you reach a sensible BMI, at which point you should feel psychologically and physically on top form. Such a regime can be classified as 'looking after yourself' rather than 'dieting'. Any desire to do things in a different, more drastic way isn't a good idea and the underlying reasons and problems need to be addressed.

Women's, admittedly sometimes tricky, relationships with food and slimming are discussed in more detail in Questions134–41 and in the last chapter.

Q130

Are there any alternative remedies or natural treatments for overeating? Can I lose weight without dieting?

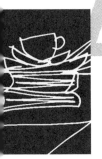

If you are asking whether you can lose weight without dieting but by taking natural herbs or going to a therapist, the answer is no. To shed weight you must create a calorie deficit so surplus fat is burnt for energy. However, there are therapies and treatments that may help the process.

Counselling to relieve stress, anxiety or depression may help by getting to the causes of overeating and/or your dependence on food. There is anecdotal evidence that acupuncture and hypnosis may help strengthen a slimming campaign and other treatments that may be of peripheral help include massage and aromatherapy, by relaxing and enhancing self-worth. Yoga and other exercise classes may also help by improving body image and resolve. Eating under Ayurvedic principles, following a Kapha-pacifying diet, may help you. A good starting point is *The Book of Ayurveda* by Judith Morrison (Gaia).

Certain Chinese herb blends may help boost weight-loss by speeding the metabolism or blunting appetite. You can also get slimming patches impregnated with scents, like vanilla, that again seem to help blunt some appetites.

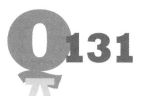 **131** **Are there slimming equivalents of one-to-one life coaches?**

Yes, you can take your pick from personal nutritionists who will help you to lose weight or from Internet diet coaches, postal diet coaches, telephone diet coaches and so on. It is very important to check out people's credentials before parting with your money, as many of these 'experts' have very little experience or expertise. Any of the top national slimming clubs may offer you more expertise and motivational help than many of these one-to-one experts.

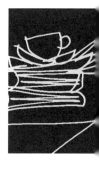

132 **Can you recommend books to help me lose weight and keep it off?**

Hopefully, this book will help you to do exactly that, but you may also find some of the following useful: *Overcoming Overeating,* Hirschmann and Hunter (Ebury Press), *Slim for Life*, Judith Wills (Vermilion), *The Food and Mood Handbook,* Amanda Geary (Thorsons), *Rosemary Conley's Low Fat Cookbook 2* (Century), *The Food Bible*, Judith Wills (Quadrille), *The Top 200 Low Fat Recipes*, Judith Wills (Headline).

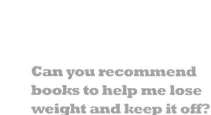

you and your life

Q133 **What are the best tips for retraining my tastebuds to enjoy healthier eating?**

This 'retraining framework' will help you re-educate your taste buds and your mind.

Start a food diary recording all you eat and drink. Using a red pen, circle everything you think contains high levels of fat (e.g. fried foods, pastry, fatty meat, dairy products), sugar (e.g. confectionery, cakes, biscuits, sweet drinks) or salt (stock cubes, packet soups/sauces, salted/cured meats, ketchup). Now, using a blue pen, circle all the following – fresh veg and fruit, fish, game and poultry, pulses, wholegrains and wholegrain products. Aim to decrease red circles and increase blue ones.

Here are some swaps to make when shopping: replace lamb shoulder with fillet, chips with new potatoes, Cheddar with Brie, fruit pie with fresh fruit. Aim to eat more fruit and veg this week – if you've been eating little, go for 1–2 portions of fruit daily and 1 of fresh veg/salad.

In the first week of such a regime, focus in particular on reducing sugar.

• Cut down its use in hot drinks and on cereal by a third, and again, 2 or 3 days later cut a few more grains, and

so on until having half what you did.
• Avoid sweet fizzy drinks, including 'diet' drinks, and use sparkling mineral water or speciality teas.
• Once or twice, have fresh fruit for dessert.
• Try to make breakfasts healthier – swap sugary cereals for non-sugared ones and add flavour with dried apricots or fresh fruit. Use natural yoghurt instead of sweetened.

After a week, go through your diary with your two pens and see if there's improvement from last week.

In the second week, focus on reducing salt. Two easy ways are to stop using salt at the table and to halve what you add in cooking. A third important way is to stop buying salty snacks and packet foods – look for 'low-salt' labels. Use fresh or dried herbs and spices for seasoning instead of salt. Also aim to reduce sugar intake a bit more – down to one-quarter of your usual quantities. Also increase further the amount of fruit and veg you have each day to 4 portions.

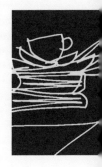

In the third week, focus on reducing fat – you will have already done this somewhat, but now consider more swaps in your daily diet.

In the fourth week, aim to:
• Omit added sugar in hot drinks, cereals, etc.
• Continue to make swaps to reduce fat, sugar and salt.
• Have 6 portions of fruit and veg daily.

At the end of the fourth week, do the red and blue pen test with the week's food diary and compare the results with week 1. Remember, your taste for food is mainly habit and can easily be altered permanently if you have the right, positive mindset.

Q134

What are eating disorders, who gets them and why?

The main eating disorders are anorexia nervosa, bulimia nervosa and binge eating disorder. Anorexia is when the person restricts the amount he/she eats and drinks far below that recommended for a normal weight-loss diet, long-term. Bulimia is when the person purges – vomiting and/or taking laxatives, to control their weight, often following bingeing and possibly starving. Binge eating disorder is long-term bouts of bingeing without purging.

People developing anorexia tend to rely on controlling food intake as a way of expressing psychological problems and/or coping with emotional difficulties. Bulimia may develop in someone who has been anorexic and may be triggered by stress.

Anyone can get an eating disorder. There are an estimated 1.15 million sufferers in the UK. Although the most common age is between 15 and 25, and there are ten female sufferers for every man, both sexes of any age can suffer. Genetic make-up may influence the chances of getting eating disorders – anorexia is eight times more likely in people with a close relative who also has

you and your life

186

anorexia, and recent research has pinpointed a gene involved in appetite control that's more frequently present in anorexics. This gene may cause the brain's food-intake mechanisms to go haywire. Also, people under strong social, parental or academic pressures may be more at risk, when the focus may shift from such pressures to food.

Major upsets – e.g. a divorce in the family, exams looming – can trigger eating disorders. Anorexia can,, though, develop because of a desire to lose weight, when normal dieting (a sensible reduced-calorie diet) becomes distorted, and bulimia can develop as a way to eat without getting fat, therefore pressure to be 'thin' is a risk factor.

The UK Eating Disorders Association says eating disorders are complex illnesses in which eating (or not) is used to block out painful feelings. There's evidence that eating disorders are 'chosen' by some and the EDA says that treatment may not always be effective if the sufferer has mixed feelings about 'giving up' their illness. Without treatment, though, problems may persist for life. Anyone with a suspected eating disorder should see a doctor.

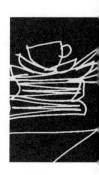

Today treatment concentrates as much, or more, on discovering and eliminating the psychological and other problems of anorexics as it does on aggressive re-feeding. The following can be contacted for help in the UK:
• Eating Disorders Association, telephone helpline for adults 0845 634 1414, helpline for under-18s 0845 634 7650. Recorded information service 0906 3020012. Website www.edauk.com
• The National Centre for Eating Disorders, tel 01372 469493, www.eating-disorders.org.uk

Q135

What are the signs of anorexia and how can it be treated?

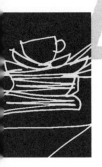

Anorexics lose weight, often to starvation levels. It may begin slowly – with a low-calorie diet, or claiming food intolerances/allergies. Eventually weight loss is extreme – they may hide this with baggy clothes, which also help protect them from cold felt because there's no fat layer.

Other symptoms are constipation, stomach pains, dizziness, fainting, swollen stomach, face and ankles, downy body hair, dry/discoloured skin, loss of periods. Psychological symptoms may include extreme fear of gaining weight, feeling they look fat not thin, mood swings and personality changes, eating rituals and enjoyment in preparing food for others, lying about what they've eaten, reluctance to eat with others, and secrecy. A recent phenomenon, termed 'orthorexia', is an obsession with 'health' foods and avoiding anything not wholesome. Orthorexics can become as dangerously thin as anorexics.

The EDA and NCfED offer help, or the sufferer and/or the family should see a GP. It's very hard for an anorexic to self-treat (they often don't agree there's a problem) and equally hard for a family to help on their own.

you and your life

188

Q 136 Will rigorous dieting make me likely to suffer from anorexia?

A It's possible, especially if you have any other 'risk factors' outlined in Question 134. Rigorous (i.e. crash) dieting – especially with long lists of forbidden foods, or rules – makes you think constantly about your diet and can make you crave forbidden foods more, or become more 'frightened' of food.

Experts tend not to think that anorexia is always – or even mostly – caused by dieting alone, because very many people lose weight without becoming anorexic and many anorexics become so without having started off with a perceived weight problem. Certainly, some cases do begin by people simply wanting to lose weight, and taking it too far, so it is best to tackle any weight-loss programme sensibly and slowly on healthy food, as outlined in this book. The ability to know when to stop is inbuilt in most people – anorexics lose this ability.

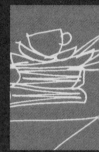

you and your life

Q137

How do I recognize someone with bulimia, why do they do this to themselves, and what should I do about it?

Bulimia nervosa means 'the hunger of an ox' and the Eating Disorders Association says that the hunger is an emotional need that can't be satisfied by food alone. Bulimia is harder to recognize than anorexia, as sufferers are often of normal weight.

A typical bulimic pattern is to binge on huge quantities of food in a short time, and then purge via vomiting and/or laxatives, and perhaps vigorous exercise. This means the food's calories aren't absorbed and the bulimic doesn't gain weight. Sometimes bulimics also alternate periods of bingeing and purging with periods of starving. Many hate themselves and fear the 'vicious circle' of bingeing and purging they can't seem to escape. Yet others use vomiting as what they see as a reasonable habit to control weight; no more socially unacceptable than smoking.

Bulimia can go undetected for years. Bulimics may appear – even to closest families – well adjusted and in control, successful and confident. However, they're often chronically lacking in self-confidence, with poor body image and emotional and psychological problems.

The most likely age to develop bulimia is between 18 and 30, and some sufferers may have had, or go on to have, anorexia. Some signs of bulimia to look out for are: fluctuating weight, disappearing to the bathroom after meals, poor skin, sore throat and hoarse voice, tooth decay (especially the teeth at the front of the mouth), general lethargy and periods of exhaustion, and sometimes periods of manic exercise. If you live with a bulimic, you may also notice food disappearing, money disappearing, empty laxative and/or diuretic packets, empty food packets in the bin, secrecy and a reluctance to enjoy social meals. Another problem with spotting bulimia in someone is that bulimics often go for months without purging. Others do it only at certain times of day.

The reason why people become bulimic is not straightforward, as there may be many factors at work and there is great variation between cases – which is why it may be difficult to spot and treat.

If you know someone with bulimia, your best course of action is probably to contact one of the eating disorder centres listed in Question 134 for advice or persuade the sufferer to visit their GP; however, the sufferer has to want to be treated and, of course, has to admit to the problem (many bulimics feel ashamed and won't admit to purging). As the Eating Disorders Association says, 'Recovery is not easy but is certainly possible.' In four out of five cases the frequency of the bouts of bingeing is reduced by therapy. Therapy can involve self-help groups, counselling, support groups, nutritional advice and more, including possibly medication, often fluoxetine (Prozac).

Q138

I'm told I'm too thin (8 stone, 5ft 7in) but I feel fat. Should I diet?

You are definitely underweight because your BMI is only just over 18. A healthy BMI is between 18.5 and 25. There's no need for you to diet any more and indeed, further dieting could be dangerous. It would be a good idea if you contact the Eating Disorders Association or the National Centre for Eating Disorders (details at the end of Question 134), or visit your doctor, as a feeling of 'fatness' when you are obviously not fat is one of the signs of anorexia.

Q139

Now and then I make myself sick for weight loss. Is this OK?

You are bulimic. There are different 'degrees' of bulimia and perhaps you're not as 'at risk' as someone who vomits or purges several times a day – but, without treatment, your occasional bouts of vomiting could easily get more frequent. Contact one of the eating disorders centres listed in Question 134 for help, as the earlier bulimia is treated the more chance you have of full recovery. If you are not convinced that 'mild' bulimia is a problem – read Questions 134–141.

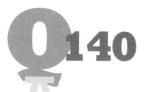

Q140 I often eat masses, like 3 whole cakes. Do I have a disorder?

If you don't purge yourself through vomiting, laxatives, etc. you seem to be a compulsive eater, with what is now called Binge Eating Disorder (see Question 134). The main symptom is weight gain, and I strongly recommend that you do seek help for your problem as soon as possible.

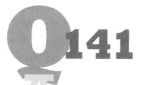

Q141 Is 'night bingeing' an eating disorder?

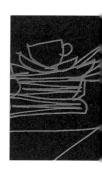

'Night eating syndrome' is an eating/sleeping disorder. Its symptoms are waking with uncontrollable feelings of hunger and cravings for carbohydrates during the night, and lack of hunger in the mornings.

Estimates are that up to a quarter of obese people may suffer from this syndrome and 1.5% of the UK population is affected. At the moment, there is no universal cure, although sufferers may benefit from counselling and a low-GI diet (see Question 66), including a low-GI snack before bed, which may help keep blood sugar levels even in the small hours and thus help prevent symptoms. Stress and a hectic lifestyle may make the problem worse.

you and your life

193

Fact one: all eating takes a certain amount of time – whether it is 'fattening' food or 'slimming' food. If you are overweight, I expect you have been finding time to eat, even though you're very busy. Fact two: high-fat, high-sugar snacks, such as chocolate and cakes, are easier and quicker to eat than items such as fresh fruit or wholegrains, even though they contain many more calories. So, I guess you have been 'filling up' on the quick-and-easy items that are the 'fattening' ones, and ignoring the healthier items.

If you want to lose weight it isn't necessary to spend a lot of time and effort on buying and eating a special or complicated diet. You just need to replace the high-fat and/or high-sugar, highly refined calorific foods with different, equally easy ones that will fill you up for fewer calories but won't take more than an extra few minutes to eat.

You can eat ready-prepared main meal salads (which come complete with fork), ready-to-eat chilled soups, ready-in-an-instant pasta with ready-made tomato or vegetable toppings, ready-washed and trimmed green salads, ready-cooked chilled chicken, ready-cooked prawns, decent bread... I could go on. For snacks, you can eat bananas, apples, nectarines. A read through the rest of this section will give you hundreds of ideas for reduced-calorie eating.

What you need to do is a one-off research session, to see what you can get without spending a lot of time shopping... supermarkets on the Internet... home box schemes... local delivery services... and to make a long list of quick and easy foods that you will enjoy without having to cook. A once-weekly, 10-minute session should then be all you need to get the week's food organized. If you really do want to lose weight, you can find this time. And if you really can't, I think you should do some serious rethinking about your priorities – the health of your body should be number one.

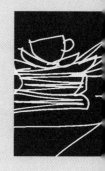

Which brings me on to the last point – it IS worth spending a few more minutes actually eating your food, as all research shows that food eaten at a slower pace satisfies you more for less calories. And it IS worth trying to eat healthily as, again, research shows that people's bodies AND brains work better when they are getting all the nutrients they need for health. You may thus save time.

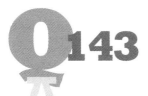

Q143

I sleep only 4 hours a night – do I burn more calories than most?

You have about 4 extra hours of activity on top of your BMR (see Question 2). Depending how you spend these, you could burn a lot more calories. If you just watch TV you'd burn only about another 30 calories an hour, totalling 120 extra. If you went walking, however, you'd burn many more. Even asleep, you burn about 60 calories an hour. However, New York's Obesity Research Centre found people who get 4 hours or less sleep nightly are 73% more likely to be obese. This appears to be because short sleep directly affects chemicals controlling weight.

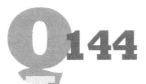

Q144

Does mental activity burn calories?

Energy is needed for your brain to function. However, there's little research on how many extra calories your brain might use in a particularly busy period of activity. The difference between reading a light novel and working flat-out all day may not amount to many calories. The proof is that sedentary people who do a great deal of hard brain work tend to get fat because they're not physically active. It's the moving parts of the body that burn most calories.

Q145 Does stress burn calories?

Quite commonly people under stress do lose weight. This can be for a variety of reasons. Stress can easily diminish appetite in the short term (e.g. the looming exam, the speech to give) and it isn't unknown for people under severe stress to lose up to a stone in a fortnight. However, for some people stress seems to increase appetite, especially for 'comfort' foods like carbohydrates.

Stress can also increase the metabolic rate – hormones released at times of stress make the heart beat faster; and stress can also make people more 'fidgety' – almost literally living off 'nervous energy'. Stress may also hasten the passage of food through the digestive system and gut, and that may then mean that less of it is actually absorbed.

However, long-term stress can also make you fat – for more on this, see Question 4 – and there is some evidence that dieters under stress tend to 'comfort eat' more. In any case, I wouldn't recommend a dose of stress as a good way of losing weight – there are too many drawbacks.

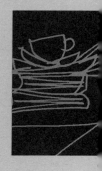

you and your life

Q146 Does smoking keep you slim?

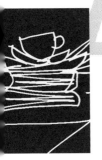

The World Health Organization says that tobacco smoking causes a 'marked' increase in the metabolic rate in the short term and may also cause a long-term increase in the basal metabolic rate. Although not all research has come to this conclusion, the evidence is quite strong, as smoking and weight gain are inversely related and smokers almost always put on weight once they give up tobacco.

Apart from the metabolism-boosting effects, people who smoke may also be slimmer because food intake is reduced. This is partly because the physical act of smoking replaces the physical act of eating and partly because smoking can suppress the appetite. However, all health authorities agree that smoking should not be used as a means to weight control, as the adverse health implications from smoking are so great.

Q147

I've given up smoking – is weight gain inevitable?

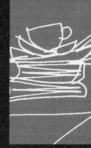

One research paper reported that the average weight gained in people who gave up smoking was 2.8kg in men and 3.8kg in women. People who smoked more than 15 cigarettes a day and then gave up tended to put on more weight and were at a higher risk of weight gain.

This weight gain is probably partly due to a slowing of the metabolic rate (see the previous question) and to an increase in appetite; because the act of eating is a substitute for the act of smoking, total calorie intake is increased.

The consensus is that the relatively small gain in weight should not be a reason to carry on smoking. I know many people who have given up smoking and have managed to keep to within two or three pounds of their 'smoking' weight. Many people who quit smoking do so because they want to have a healthier lifestyle. Once the lungs are free from tobacco pollution, exercising becomes a much more viable option – and so ex-smokers can easily, and often do, reset their metabolism to a higher rate via regular exercise.

you and your life

Q148 Can you give me some ideas for quick and/or easy, non-fattening but delicious suppers for 1 or 2 people?

It is easier than you might think, especially if you eat meat and fish, as the supermarkets have so many quick-cooking low-fat choices. Think fairly small portions, bulked out with lots of vegetables (again there are so many ready-prepared ones to choose from) and some decent-quality carbohydrate (new potatoes, rice, noodles, pasta, couscous, bulgar are all cheap, quick and easy).

The griddle or frying pan is, of course, a boon for quick after-work cooking, and I never mind cooking with a little olive oil or a small dab of butter for the main meal of the day – as long as you mostly avoid the obviously calorific foods like pastry, and save things like double cream for special occasions, you can't go far wrong.

The following after-work meals each serve 2 and contain around 500 calories a portion; 15g ($\frac{1}{2}$oz) fat max:
• 100g ($3\frac{1}{2}$oz) (dry weight) wholewheat pasta topped with a seafood sauce made by simmering good-quality ready-made pasta tomato sauce with 200g (7oz) defrosted mixed frozen seafood and some sliced mushrooms and fresh basil; salad.

• 2 medium turkey escalopes, fried in a non-stick pan with low-calorie cooking oil spray, served with 100g (3½oz) (dry weight) rice noodles, cooked; and stir-fry of mixed frozen vegetables with a dessertspoon of yellow bean sauce and 2 tablespoons chicken stock.

• 2 medium salmon fillets brushed with good-quality ready-made pesto sauce, grilled and served with ready-prepared baby new potatoes or wild rice; broccoli.

• 100g (3½oz) (dry weight) basmati rice, cooked with a good pinch of ground curry spices; mixed with 150g (5oz) smoked haddock fillet, microwaved and flaked, and 75g (2¾oz) cooked peas; with a poached egg each on top.

• Large bowl of mixed salad leaves, tossed with 4 slices extra-lean back bacon grilled; dressing of 1 tablespoon olive oil and 1 dessertspoon balsamic vinegar, 1 teaspoon wholegrain mustard, seasoning; crusty roll each.

• 2 chicken breasts, skinned, cubed and skewered, brushed with yoghurt mixed with crushed garlic; grilled and served with lemons, 50g (1⅔oz) (dry weight) couscous, reconstituted; tomato and red onion salsa.

• 300g (10½oz) pork fillet, sliced and stir-fried with ready-prepared carrot batons and broccoli and halved spring onions, 1 tablespoon sesame oil, soy sauce, and ready-prepared ginger, plus 2 tablespoons chicken stock; serve with 50g (1⅔oz) (dry weight) egg noodles.

• 2 medium fresh mackerel fillets, grilled and served with a sauce of Greek yoghurt mixed with horseradish sauce, baby spinach microwaved in its own pack and ready-prepared baby new potatoes.

See also Questions 103, 106, 116, 151 and 172–4.

you and your life

Is it OK to diet on nothing but convenience foods?

Everyone makes use of such things as microwave meals for one now and then, and they are a boon – but when choosing, do read the label and make sure that it doesn't contain more than about 15g of fat per serving. This will mean that you can have about 15g fat for lunch, and a little fat in your breakfast and daily snacks without going over a daily 42g total fat, which will give you a 25% fat diet for an average woman slimming on 1,500 calories a day.

Also, try to find ready meals that contain plenty of vegetables. Otherwise, add a pack of mixed salad leaves to your basket and eat a big side salad too. Most ready meals also contain the 'carbohydrate' element of the meal (rice, pasta, etc.). If so (for females with an average metabolic rate slimming on 1,500 calories a day), you can afford to choose a meal up to 500 calories. If yours doesn't, make sure that it's no more than around 300 calories a serving, so that you can add some carbohydrate of your own at home – the simplest would be about 50g (1²⁄₃ oz) of wholemeal bread or roll.

you and your life

Meals like beans on toast are also fine sometimes – the pulses are very healthy and the tomato sauce is a good source of lycopene; make the bread wholemeal and it's a very good meal, low in fat unless you add lots of butter to your toast. I'd add an orange afterwards, otherwise you won't get any vitamin C. This will also help the body absorb the iron in the beans and bread.

If you choose very carefully, varying your choices, you may well be fine nutritionally on a diet of convenience foods and things on toast, especially if you add fresh fruit and salad. However, one of the main disadvantages of many of the ready meals is that you don't get very much on your plate – many slimmers could eat TWO portions easily! So without high satiety value, you may feel hungry and increase the amount of food you eat in snacks between meals. Some are not all that tasty or exciting, either, although some brands are quite good. Also be aware that recent research shows nutritional information on the packets of convenience foods can be as much as 20% 'out' – i.e. if the pack says a portion contains 300 calories, for instance, it could actually contain 360.

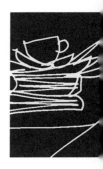

Convenience meals in a pack are saving you time and trouble – but check out the other ideas in this section of the book and you'll see that there are many simple main meals and lunches that you can prepare almost as quickly from scratch. If you have a wide variety of foods and tastes on your slimming plan you're more likely to stick with it and succeed.

Assuming you are one of the many people who work late, then call into a takeaway on the way home – there are some items you could choose which would be better for your waistline, but the trouble is that, in my experience, you will be so hungry that caution goes out the window and you choose the most calorific thing you can see on the menu – plus, of course, there are all the food aromas as you order, to get your taste buds going!

This is one of the trickiest problems to solve. It would be best if you could adjust your schedule or, failing that, have something nice but not so calorific in your briefcase or bag that you can eat during your last hour at work – say, a small ham sandwich or even a bag of low-fat crisps. This will take the edge off your appetite and then you could wait until you get home, where you can heat up a (decent-quality) ready meal or cook a quick steak or bowl of pasta – or reheat something you made earlier, perhaps.

The thing about losing weight is that you have to be committed, and you have to plan. If what you eat is last on your list of priorities, of course you are going to have problems. You have to decide what is most important to you. Hopefully you'll decide that you do want to lose weight and feel good about your diet, in which case you may like to invest an hour or so at weekends in making a few simple things for the freezer (assuming you're very busy all week). If you're not short of cash and live in a city, you can probably even find companies via the Internet who will bike you round a healthy meal to order.

A fairly short list of takeaway meals that can be fitted into most slimming plans includes sushi, tandoori chicken, vegetable chilli with rice, vegetable or seafood lasagne, and jacket potato with beans or sweetcorn and tuna. Sadly, however, very many takeout foods – including most of the menu in Indian, Chinese, Thai, Mexican, pizza houses, burger bars, chicken bars, fish and chip shops – ARE full of fat and therefore high in calories and best saved for occasional use. A list of common takeaways with their calorie and fat values appears in Question 101.

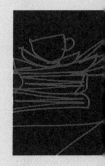

TIP: One of the most important things to remember for very busy people is to eat 'little and often' throughout the day, to keep blood sugar levels even and stop you from wanting to 'pig out' the minute you stop work and realize you're ravenous.

Q151

Shiftworkers sometimes get in a muddle with set diets because some days – particularly when shift hours change – they may have an extra meal, or two main meals, instead of a breakfast and main meal. Shiftworkers also tend to snack on high-fat items, like chocolate and biscuits.

If that's what is bothering you, the best way to cope is first to understand that losing weight doesn't necessarily mean sticking to three set meals a day in strict order and, second, that to avoid getting very hungry and snacking on chocolate, etc. you need to plan ahead a little.

If you can lose weight on 1,500 calories a day (most people can), in theory you could divide these calories up any way you want over any 24-hour period. As 'little and often' is best for health and will also suit your lifestyle, you could divide it into, say, four mini-meals a day of 300 calories each (and have the extra for milk, drinks, treats).

It's best to stick with mini-meals that are easy to eat and quick to prepare, Another tip is to choose things that can serve as breakfast, lunch, supper, whatever. It's also best to take your food to work with you, if the only

you and your life

206

alternative will be a badly stocked cafeteria – when working nights, buying decent food is always a problem.

You could keep a weekly food diary, each day divided into four spaces into which you write what you've eaten as soon as is practical. That way, at the end of the week you can see how many of your mini-meals you've had. Even if one or two extra show, you should still lose weight slowly. On days when you want to sleep all day to 'catch up', perhaps there will be fewer meals to record, anyway.

Mini-meal ideas – each about 300 calories:

• Calorie-counted (250 or less) ready-to-eat sandwich; piece of fruit.

• Big bowl of ready-to-eat, chilled-counter vegetable soup with 1 small slice of bread.

• Bowl of wholegrain cereal with skimmed milk and fresh and dried chopped fruit.

• 150g (5oz) baked beans on 40g (1⅓oz) toast.

• Ready-cooked chicken breast portion with side salad and small roll.

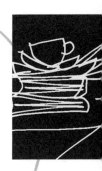

• 2 small eggs, poached, on wholemeal toast with low-fat spread; 1 satsuma.

• Breakfast bowl of cooked pasta, topped with ready-made Italian tomato sauce and a little grated Parmesan.

• 200g (7oz) baked potato topped with 50g (1⅔oz) baked beans and 20g (⅔oz) grated Parmesan.

• 200g (7oz) cooked basmati rice mixed with chopped chicken, salad veg and pine nuts, with oil-free dressing.

If this 'four meals a day' idea doesn't appeal, just do your own thing. If your weekly calorie total gives you an energy deficit, how you ate those calories doesn't matter.

you and your life

207

Q152 I haven't time for breakfast and I prefer to have my main meal late in the evening. Can this cause weight gain?

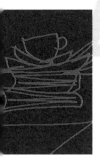

As Question 80 explains, it is the total number of calories you eat in a day (or week) that is more important than when you eat them as a deciding factor in whether or not you gain weight. As long as you aren't taking in more calories over a period of time than you are burning off in activity/energy then you shouldn't put on weight eating this way.

However most experts agree that a small healthy breakfast is a good idea after the long night's fast (Question 79) and some research shows that people who prefer morning eating to evening eating consume many fewer calories over the course of the day.

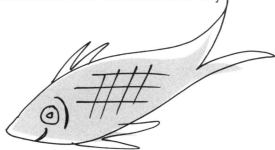

Q153

Most working people have lunch around 1pm – and seven hours is too long to go without eating anything. Matters are compounded if you have to spend an hour in the kitchen after work preparing a meal – of course you'll pick, it's only natural.

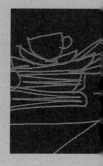

What you need to do is have an 'allowed' snack when you get home – around 100–200 calories. If this contains foods low on the Glycaemic Index (see Question 66), then it should keep hunger at bay until 8. Some suggestions are: 2 dark rye crispbreads topped with Marmite and slices of tomato (80 calories); 1 individual tub of diet fruit yoghurt and an apple (130 calories); 1 heaped tbsp reduced-fat hummus on 1 mini pitta (130 calories).

To make amends for this, give yourself slightly smaller portions of other meals throughout the day – to reduce any meal by 50 calories you only have to serve yourself, say, 30g (1oz) less meat or half a slice of bread less.

Another solution you could incorporate is to have half your lunch at 1pm and the remainder at 2 or 3, if possible (or have lunch later).

you and your life

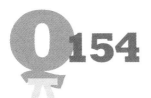

Q154 How do I resist the coffee and snacks trolley at work?

If you know when it comes, the best bet is to make sure you have had a small healthy snack just before it arrives – you can easily fit two such snacks a day into you diet. Snack suggestions appear in the answer to the previous question.

Q155 I travel a lot and eat at pubs and cafés. What can I do to slim?

The best idea would be to take an insulated lunchbox with you, filled with tempting lower-fat foods and snacks (Question 159 will help here). You can pull off the road for half an hour – and probably save yourself time as well.

If this isn't possible, stock up in the supermarket with ready-made, calorie-counted sandwiches, wraps, sushi or other 'healthy options' lunch foods.

Also bear in mind that when you are at home and in control of what you eat is the time to major on low-calorie, very healthy meals, plenty of veg and so on.

Skipping lunch isn't ideal for most people, as blood sugar levels will begin to dip without anything to eat since breakfast. As a compromise, you could have a reasonably large breakfast, including items low on the Glycaemic Index (see Question 66) and take to work a couple of portable snacks to eat at quiet moments during your working day – ideally, one at around 12 noon and the other around 3.30pm. Two 150-calorie snacks would be ideal, again, with a low GI, which will help keep your blood sugar levels stable until you have your meal.

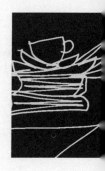

As I have said before, how much you eat is what counts in maintaining or losing weight. HOW and when you eat are more important for other reasons – perhaps health, convenience and helping you stick to any diet regime. What works best for you is what matters most – but for most people, skipping lunch inevitably means the (sometimes uncontrollable) urge to eat something high in calories and/or fat and/or sugar or starch in the late afternoon or early evening.

you and your life

Q157

Our cafeteria majors on pies, chips, sausage, etc. – or quiche and salad or things on toast. What's the best bet, calorie-wise?

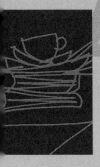

Take your own lunch to work! Seriously, most of the things you mention are high in fat and best avoided on anything except an occasional basis. A quiche salad is much higher in fat and calories than you would think, because of the pastry, egg and salad dressing, and is probably no better than sausage and chips. Cheese and biscuits are also high in fat and high density, meaning that you don't get much on your plate, and there are no vegetables or salad with this, either.

If taking your own lunch to work isn't feasible, is there anywhere else locally you could go for a more slimmer-friendly lunch? Otherwise, I'd find out who is responsible for the menu at your company cafeteria and see if you can get them to put at least one 'healthy option' on the menu each day. If they aren't helpful, go to your company boss and ask them instead. The list of fast foods shown in Question 101 may help you make the best choices from what is currently on offer.

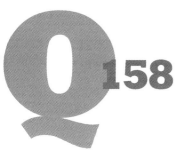

Q158

There's no simple solution, but several tactics may help you to cut down on surplus calories. If being entertained, avoid pre-meal nibbles, or take just one or two, if offered. During the meal, say no to extras like bread, butter, spring rolls, etc. If self-service is called for, give yourself small portions. If offered seconds, refuse politely. Most hostesses the world over don't mind if you refuse dessert. And say no also to any chocolates or other titbits with coffee.

Alcohol is easy – just say you're not drinking at the moment. If you can't bear the thought of avoiding all alcohol, just take the first drink and have it slowly. For more tips on alcohol avoidance see Question 169.

If on your own in the hotel, simply order the plainest things you can find: grilled steak, fish or chicken, salad, new potatoes. On a plane there are usually fewer calories in airline meals than you might think, as portions are quite small. Just leave the roll, butter and dessert.

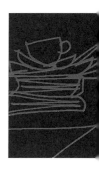

you and your life

213

Q159

Can you give me ideas for healthy low-fat lunchbox meals for adults?

Very many sandwiches, filled rolls, wraps, etc. are quite low in fat and calories. If making up your own lunchbox, simply choose decent-quality bread, a low-fat protein filling (e.g. lean ham, chicken, turkey, tuna, prawns) or occasionally a medium-fat filling (egg, Brie), add plenty of salad items, dress with a little low-fat mayonnaise (or nothing) and there you are. Pittas are great – easily stuffed with feta and salad or tuna and salad, or buy your own wraps and roll them up with more exotic fillings – chicken and pesto, seafood and chilli. If buying sandwiches, simply look for the words 'low-fat' and/or 'low-calorie'.

You will want to add other items to the pack: always choose a piece of fresh fruit and then pick one (or possibly two, depending upon your metabolic rate and dieting level) more item(s) from: individual tubs of yoghurt or fromage frais, a small bag filled with some ready-to-eat dried fruit and fresh nuts or pumpkin seeds, malt loaf, tea bread, plain scone, good-quality fruit cake.

If you get bored with all bready-things, think about sushi, or various lunch salads, which you can pack in a little box and eat with plastic fork! You can buy several ready-made, but here are ideas for salads to make at home.

• Couscous and Red Pepper: 50g (1²/₃oz) (dry weight) couscous, reconstituted in vegetable stock and mixed with grilled, sliced peppers, basil leaves, 25g (³/₄oz) halloumi, chopped, and 1 tablespoon olive oil vinaigrette (400 calories)

• New Potato and Egg Salad: 175g (6oz) cold cooked new potatoes, roughly chopped and mixed with 1 medium hard-boiled egg, chopped, 1 slice of lean back bacon, grilled and crumbled, 50g (1²/₃oz) small cooked broad beans, wedges of Little Gem lettuce and 1 tablespoon dijonnaise dressing mixed with 1 tablespoon low-fat natural bio yoghurt and seasoning (375 calories).

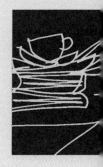

• Rice and Bean Salad: 150g (5oz) (cooked weight) basmati rice mixed with 100g (3¹/₂oz) cooked mixed pulses (well drained) OR chickpeas, 3 pieces ready-to-eat dried apricot, chopped, 1 tablespoon pine nuts, chopped celery and cucumber and oil-free French dressing to taste (375 calories).

• Pasta and Tuna Salad: 150g (5oz) (cooked weight) wholewheat pasta shapes mixed with 100g (3¹/₂oz) flaked bluefin tuna in water, well drained, 25g (³/₄oz) cooked sweetcorn kernels, chopped tomato, parsley, cucumber and oil-free French dressing to taste (300 calories).

Add a bottle of mineral water or a flask of tea – most drinks add too many calories to your lunch for little benefit and low-cal fizzy drinks just encourage a sweet tooth. In warm weather, or warm offices, take your lunch in an insulated lunchbox/bag – these are now widely available.

you and your life

Q160

Are there any snacks, like peanuts and crisps, which are just as tempting but not so fattening?

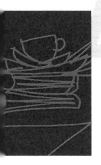

You can buy several brands of reduced-fat, reduced-calorie crisps and savoury snacks – in the UK, Boots do a good 'Shapers' range, with every pack under 100 calories. Other brands include WeightWatchers Weavers, KP Skips, Golden Wonder Lites. Popcorn is another good idea – it is filling and reasonable healthy, and a small bag will satisfy you at around 115 calories. Pretzels and Twiglets are both fairly low in calories, too, but make sure to buy small packs, and remember lots of savoury snacks are high in salt.

Another good idea for home use is to buy fresh nuts in their shells, and crack them open yourself. Not only are the nuts healthy, tasty, salt-free and good for you, but if you have to crack them it will slow down your rate of eating to a quarter your usual rate. Yes, nuts are high in calories, but only if you eat too many of them!

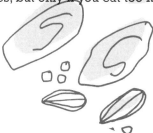

Q 161

I'm entertained in restaurants at least 3 lunches and 2 evenings a week, which has made me gain weight. How do I cope with this?

Assuming that you can pick your own menu from what is on offer, the next question offers plenty of tips on reducing the total calorie content of your meal without seeming to be a spoilsport.

Other tips for not offending your host appear in Question 163. Much of the etiquette when being entertained in restaurants is exactly the same as that expected when being entertained in private homes.

I should also point out that if you have three lunches and two evenings out each week that also leaves four lunches and five evenings when you can control your diet. Going on the swings-and-roundabouts principle, perhaps at these times you could be a bit harder on yourself. It is the overall number of calories you consume that counts, not the total in any one particular meal.

Also, try to take some extra exercise if you know you've had a particularly calorific week.

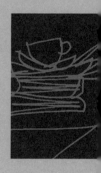

Of course, hotel menus will vary depending on where you are in the world but, assuming 'international' standard hotels, choices can be remarkably similar. If dining alone, just have a main course – this will immediately bring your calorie total down to a reasonable level. Choose anything grilled or roasted – fish and chicken being a good bet. Tenderloin of pork is a very lean hotel favourite. Lamb often comes with a fair amount of fat still attached, so perhaps is best avoided.

Sauces can add a lot of fat and calories to your meal, so choose wisely. 'Mediterranean'-style sauces based on tomato are fine, though they may be high in olive oil. 'Meunière' means butter – these and rich cream sauces are ones to pass on, or have in very small amounts, as are béchamel, au gratin, and hollandaise. Ask the waiter for your meal without the sauce, or for the sauce served separately so you can put just a dab on, if necessary. Also ask if you aren't sure what a dish contains in the way of butter, oil or cream.

Definitely ask for your side vegetables to come

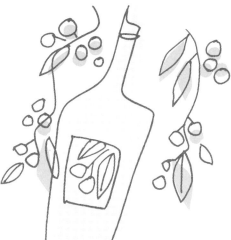

without butter garnish, skip the bread (or at least the
butter with the bread). You can also save lots of calories
by asking for rice cooked plain and for new or baked
potato rather than roast or chips. You may prefer to stick
with the protein and vegetable element of the meal and
skip the starch (potatoes, pasta, bread, rice). This isn't a
particularly healthy way to eat, but it is a fairly simple
way of keeping the calories down (but not the fat).

Some ethnic main courses will be fine, but there isn't
room here to second-guess all that you may be offered.
Hotel 'help yourself' buffets are useful but, for the
unwary, some of the salads on offer are very high in fat.
If they are 'glistening', they are probably thick with
mayonnaise or oil.

For dessert, if you're being wise you'll stick with fruit
salad or fresh fruit platter.

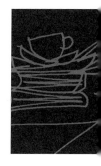

Q 163 I am often invited to dinner in people's homes, where there's no choice. How do I eat fewer calories without causing offence?

There's nothing worse than turning up for a carefully prepared dinner and announcing you're on a diet. I know people do it but, unless there is medical reason, it seems obsessive. If you know the host well, have a word beforehand and say you're trying to lose a few pounds (on doctor's orders, if you like) and so he/she isn't to feel offended if you have smaller portions and may refuse dessert. If you don't know the host well, follow the tips below. However, for anyone who dines out rarely, an occasional evening's overindulgence isn't going to make a great deal of difference to your total calorie input in the long term, so perhaps it's best to sit back and enjoy it!

• Avoid more than one canapé. No one will notice.
• Avoid crisps and other high-fat savoury nibbles left out in bowls – they ruin your appetite for the meal, anyway. Again, no one will notice whether you eat these or not.
• Sip drinks very slowly, putting your glass down between sips. If you're driving, you have the excuse not to drink.
• Don't take bread or butter – this won't offend the host.
• If food arrives 'self-service', take only small portions of

the high-calorie items. If there are several people present, no one is likely to notice. You could even pass on the sautéed potatoes or the like without causing comment.

• If your host dishes food out herself/himself at the table, when you're being given yours, smile and say, 'That's lovely, thank you,' before she/he gets a chance to dish too much out.

• If seconds are offered, decline gracefully.

• Many hosts don't feel offended if you skip dessert– if yours insists, it is fine to ask for a small portion. If there is a choice, avoid the rich, creamy dessert and go for the fruit.

• Avoid the cheeseboard and after-dinner chocolates, etc.

Also bear in mind that going out once or even twice at weekends, and eating a bit more than you would have done at home, aren't the end of the world for your diet – it leaves all week to be more restrained. A supper or dinner party is to be enjoyed – not something that makes you feel guilty. A long walk the next day helps, too.

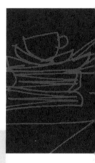

Party nibble calories

Piece of salmon sushi – 50
Breadstick – 20
Mini chicken kiev – 50
One carrot crudité and
  cheese dip – 25
Mini pizza (2 mouthfuls) – 100
Breaded prawn – 40
Baked potato wedge with dip – 45
Won ton – 35
Individual quiche (2 bites) – 100

Red pepper slice and
  salsa dip – 10
Cocktail sausage – 40
Hummus/roast veg crostini – 50
Mini samosa – 80
New potato with sour cream
  topping – 60
Chicken vol au vent
  (2 mouthfuls) – 80
Marinated olive – 5

you and your life

221

Q164

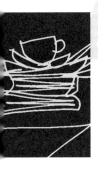

Certainly this is one way to cut calories when eating out, and for people who are unsure which choices are high-calorie or high-fat and which aren't, it is a fairly simple and foolproof way of doing so. If you just avoid the potatoes, rice, pasta, bread, couscous and so on, you will save on average about 300–400 calories on the total meal. If you love meat, for example, you may like to do this.

You could probably, however, save more if instead you deliberately go for items very low in fat, and take the plainly cooked carbohydrate items such as new potatoes or plain boiled rice. This is also, long-term, a healthier way of eating – though going the low-carb route now and then won't do you any harm.

Q165

When eating out, on balance is it best to have a starter and main course or a main course and dessert ?

You can choose starters that are quite low in calories and you can also choose desserts that are quite low in calories, so it's a matter of personal preference. The other questions in this section will point you towards good choices and steer you away from the less good.

There may be something to be said for having a starter, as it will take the edge off your appetite and you may be less inclined to overeat on your main course. It is also the thing to go for if you are following a high-protein, low-carbohydrate diet.

Also, in some restaurants it is quite hard to find a dessert that is on the 'good' rather than the 'less good' list. So my inclination would be to go for the starter. On the other hand, if you love desserts, when the dessert menu is handed round you will need an iron will to refuse, even if you have had a starter!

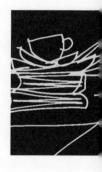

you and your life

Q166

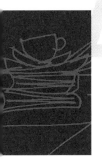

Fresh fruit, fruit salads and sorbets are the absolutely blameless desserts, while several others come 'in the balance', for example ice cream, meringue and zabaglione. Anything with a lot of pastry, cream and/or chocolate and anything laden with mascarpone cheese are all very high in calories, fat and sugar. If you only eat out once in a blue moon, however, I don't see why you shouldn't have what you feel like, and perhaps cut back a bit on your calorie and fat intake the following day.

I would say that a 'good' or a 'reasonable' dessert would definitely be a better bet, with respect to calories and fat, than the cheeseboard. If you choose cheese (much of which will be high in fat, calories and saturated fat), you will also be offered butter and fat-rich crackers, oatcakes, etc. If you are a 'cheeseaholic' and really do want to try the cheeses, I suggest you plan for this: skip the starter and have a very low-fat main course, then you can eat your cheese without feeling guilty.

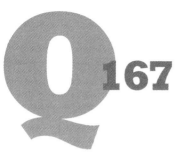

Q167

Because I eat out a lot, I don't want the restriction of a 'set diet'. Any guidelines to make sure I lose weight?

I think your best bet is to follow the 'traffic light' system outlined in Question 95. If you are sensible and don't cheat, this should produce steady weight loss without any calorie or fat counting, or any other fiddly methods of weight loss. You might also consider trying a high-protein/low-carbohydrate diet. It's not as healthily balanced as a good healthy-eating diet should be, but it does achieve results.

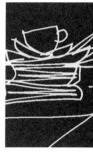

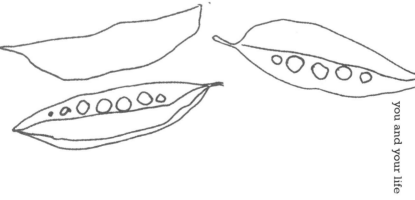

Q168

I eat sensibly but drink a bottle of wine every evening. Is this the cause of my steady weight gain?

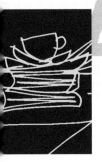

A bottle of wine has 500–600 calories and that on top of a normal day's food intake, could put on roughly a pound a week. If weight gain's been slower, you're probably eating a little less to 'allow' for the wine. However, it's hard to stay slim when drinking more than a glass or two nightly.

The average female needs about 2,000 calories a day to maintain weight. A bottle of wine equals at least 500, so in order not to gain weight you can only have 1,500 food calories. It's easy to go over this. You'd also need to be diligent in getting vitamins, minerals, etc. in your food, as wine contains no major nutrients except alcohol and sugar.

Also, a bottle of wine a day is double that recommended for a female – you could also be setting yourself up for health problems. The next question should help you cut intake by at least half. You don't have to give up wine completely, but more than a glass or two daily is hard to fit into a slimming diet without nutritional balance suffering.

Q169

What tips do you have for cutting down on alcohol? I have to attend a lot of drinks parties and I drink most days.

A First you have to get into the right 'mindset' – you really need to want to reduce your alcohol intake. The following tips should help:

• Drive to parties, so you can say you're driving.

• Have a pint of water before drinking – thirst can make you drink more than you need.

• Alternate one alcoholic drink with a soft drink, or mix wine with equal parts soda water for a spritzer.

• Sip drinks slowly and put your glass down when you can. If a waiter approaches with a bottle, be strong and turn your back.

• Single measures of spirits with low-cal mixers are a better bet than wine for many people. A single measure contains only 50 calories and one alcohol unit, while an average glass (150ml/ $\frac{1}{4}$ pint) of 12.5% strength wine contains 2 units and about 100 calories.

• Remember, it's your life – drink (sensibly) if you want to, but not if you don't.

• As a substitute for wine, try 'adult' cordials, like elderflower, nettle and citrus, mixed with ice-cold water.

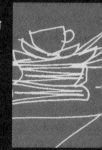

you and your life

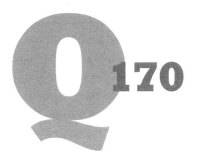

Q170

I have a family of ravenous children and cook a lot, but find I'm tempted to nibble while cooking; have you any tips for breaking this habit?

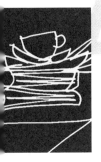

Ensure you're not ravenous while preparing food. Eat 'little and often' during the day so that you never reach the 'ravenous' stage, choosing foods and snacks low on the Glycaemic Index (Question 66). Even if trying to lose weight, you shouldn't ever need to feel starving.

Also, keep a container of things to eat while preparing food – say crudités with fat-free dip, or dark rye crispbread spread with Marmite. These will add very little to your day's calorie or fat tally and will keep you happy while you cook.

It's difficult to avoid tasting anything while you cook and is not how cooks operate. If you frequently cook your family something you love and feel won't fit in with your diet, however, you make life harder for yourself. If that happens often, perhaps rethink what you're feeding the family. Should they need many more calories than you do, perhaps you could cook 'healthy' for them and simply increase their portion sizes and add extra starch items, such as bread and potatoes. It's always a good idea to get your children keen on lean meats, fish, veg and grains.

Q171

How can I stop myself from eating the food I buy for the children's lunchboxes – cakes and so on?

Your wanting to eat the children's cakes suggests to me that you are suffering from fluctuating blood sugar levels, probably because you're trying to diet and not eating often enough, and/or of foods low on the GI (see the previous question).

You will be tempted to eat sugary items if you get back from the shops, unpack the food and notice cake when your blood sugar levels are low. Eat a low-GI food before you go shopping and have a ready-prepared snack waiting in the fridge for you when you get in.

Don't try to diet on too few calories – check your metabolic rate and your proper dieting calorie intake. Also consider giving your children more items in their lunchboxes which perhaps you won't feel too guilty about 'pinching' – fruit, dried fruit, fresh nuts, seeds, good-quality fruit cake rather than sugary sponges, lower-fat crisps and so on. It's good to help them grow up with less of a sweet (and salty) tooth than you have yourself. Take a look at the retraining framework in Question 133.

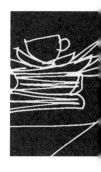

you and your life

Q172 I can't afford to diet – how are poor people expected to buy '5 a day', for example? I've only £15 a week to spend on food. Any advice?

One of the best ways to save money on fruit and veg is by buying in bulk, but that's probably not an option unless you can organize a co-op with like-minded neighbours. Even then, if you live alone you may not be able to store the food. Let's look at ways you can eat to slim (and get your 5 a day) without spending over your limit.

First of all, although '5 a day' is a good idea for you, it isn't essential for successful slimming. Even if you manage 2–4 portions a day, you'll be doing better than many people. However, eating more fruit and vegetable does help a slimming diet by 'bulking up' plates for few calories, so here are ways to work some into your low-cost diet.

• Pulses – baked beans, butter beans, red kidney beans, lentils, etc. – all count towards veg intake and are among the lowest-cost foods. See the previous question for tips. They are also low in fat and calories, high in fibre and low-GI, to keep you feeling full, and have an almost perfect balance of protein and carbohydrate.

• Although it doesn't taste as good as fresh, long-life

orange juice is a good and inexpensive source of vitamin C and will keep well for several days, even when opened (in the fridge).

• Fresh fruits that tend to be cheapest are apples, bananas, kiwi fruits and satsumas. Buy whichever is the least expensive at the time and enough for the week – one a day. Kiwi and satsumas are highest in vitamin C, but apples are good for the blood and bananas a great source of energy. You could afford seven pieces of fruit a week at an average of 15p a piece.

• Basic vegetables in season – such as cabbage, greens, carrots, onions, swede – should be fairly inexpensive and you could buy one portion a day for about 20p. Other veg may also be cheap at times and/or may be on special offer.

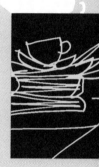

• If you do have a freezer, or a freezer compartment to your fridge, large packs of peas or sweetcorn kernels can be a good buy. A portion is about 3 tablespoons (80g/3oz) and a 1 kilo (2lb) pack will last you for about 12 meals. This works out at about 16p a portion. Both are high in fibre and vitamin C and fairly low in calories.

• For other cost-saving ideas, see Questions 173 and 174.

So, you could have 1 glass of orange juice, 1 piece of fresh fruit, 1 fresh vegetable, 1 pulse and 1 frozen vegetable a day for a total cost of around 90p. As I said, you don't have to have all that – a varied choice of 3 or 4 would be acceptable, and the remainder of your cash can be spent on bread, potatoes, cereal, tea and all the other healthy items that make up a low-cost slimming diet.

you and your life

Q173

The previous and next questions will give you a general idea of which foods are low-cost and healthy, but here are a few more specific guidelines for your own situation. First look at this list of low-cost, quick-and-easy foods that can form part of your healthy slimming diet:

• Carbs: bread, dried pasta, rice, couscous, bulgar wheat, egg thread noodles, baking potatoes, breakfast cereals.

• Proteins: medium or low-fat cheeses*, such as Brie, Edam, Camembert, feta, halloumi, mozzarella, goats' cheese; extra-lean ham*, cooked turkey*, eggs, canned tuna, mackerel; baked beans and all cooked canned pulses; fresh chicken thigh portions*, skimmed milk* or buy long-life, natural yoghurt*, Greek yoghurt*.

• Fruits: fresh apples, bananas, kiwis, satsumas and other fruits in season; dried apricots and peaches, prunes, figs, raisins; canned fruits in natural juice; lemons (keep well and ideal for dressings/flavouring).

• Veg: tomatoes, lettuce, onion and cucumber (price varies on salads, but cheap for several months a year); canned tomatoes, canned peppers, white cabbage and carrot

(these both store well and are good in salads/soups).
• Miscellaneous: dried herbs and spices, seasoning, ketchup, Worcestershire sauce, soy sauce, vinegar, olive oil, stock cubes, low-fat spread*, ready-made tomato sauce for pasta, low-fat cook-in sauce for chicken, pasta or fish, Marmite, low-sugar jam, runny honey, hummus, curry powder. (* need to be stored in a fridge. If possible also store fresh fruit and veg in a fridge.)

Now here are ideas on how to make these foods into decent meals that will fill you up without piling on pounds. Take a little time to plan out what you may need for a few days ahead (if you don't have a fridge you'll have to buy any starred items that you want just before you eat them) which will save time and money in the long run:

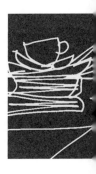

Breakfast: cereal with skimmed milk or yoghurt and fresh or dried fruit OR bread, low-fat spread and low-sugar jam, yoghurt and fruit.

Lunch: egg on toast OR lean ham and tomatoes OR leftover cooked rice salad with chopped apple, ham and apricot OR leftover couscous salad with raisins, chopped onion, carrot and cooked chicken.

Evening: baked (microwaved) potato with ready-to-eat tomato sauce and grated medium-fat cheese, e.g. Edam or mozzarella.OR stir-fry of sliced chicken thigh portions (ready-skinned and boned) stir-fried in a little oil with sliced carrot, white cabbage and onion, soy sauce and seasoning to taste. Serve with egg thread noodles. OR pasta shapes, boiled and topped with ready-to-eat tomato sauce (with basil or herbs), stirred with canned tuna.

Dessert: Greek yoghurt with honey or fresh fruit; low-fat bio yoghurt topped with muesli.

Q174

I have a tight budget and need a main meal of the day of about £1 a head for 4. Can you advise on healthy non-fattening meals that fit the bill?

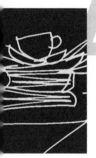

You can keep costs down by:
• Buying fruits and vegetables in season and/or locally produced and/or bulk-buying with neighbours.
• Basing several meals a week around pulses – dried pulses are cheaper than canned and only need soaking overnight, and sometimes pre-boiling. Add small bits of meat to your pulses for flavour and 'complete protein'.
• Eating less protein and more grains and potatoes – many of us eat more protein than we actually need for health. Dishes of pasta, brown rice and other low-cost grains or baked potatoes, topped with vegetables sauces and a little grated cheese, are ideal.
• Some oily fish are low-cost and very healthy – try mackerel or herring fillets grilled with seasonal vegetables, or buy them in cans for quick lunches.
• When using meat, concentrate on slow-cooking methods, like stews and casseroles, as slow-cook cuts are cheaper and often tastier. Let them cool and skim fat off before reheating (cheaper cuts are usually fattier). If you buy standard mince, pre-cook it to remove the fat.

Q175

Is it OK to cut out meat and dairy produce and save calories that way?

If you cut these out without replacing them with anything else, you'll certainly save calories (assuming you'd been eating a reasonable amount of them regularly) and will probably reduce the total fat and saturated fat in your diet. However, a read of the next question will show you that you may fall short of a variety of nutrients if you don't make an effort to replace them. So just cutting out large chunks of your diet isn't as good an idea as you may think.

If you like meat and dairy, why not simply eat less of them (and choose leaner, or less-fat varieties) and follow a varied healthy diet. If you don't like meat and dairy, you will have to ensure you get a varied diet that replaces key nutrients such as iron, calcium and protein.

Remember, any kind of fad/restricted diet is not often the best way to reduce calories. As a group, the statistics show that vegetarians are generally slimmer and healthier than meat-eaters, but other factors may be involved. For example, there are many more non-smokers amongst vegetarians, and veggies tend to take more exercise and live generally 'healthier' lives than the rest of us.

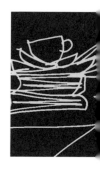

you and your life

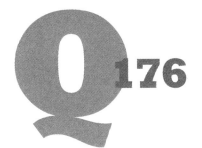

Q176 Can a vegetarian slimming diet give me all the nutrients I need?

Yes it can – but even with a normal maintenance vegetarian diet, as you're living off a more restricted diet than omnivores, you may need to try a little harder to get all your requirements. On a vegetarian slimming plan, you have to be even more vigilant about getting a healthy range of foods, because you are eating less and there is thus potentially more chance for shortfalls of nutrients.

If you are following a reduced-calorie diet without meat, poultry or fish, the nutrients that you are most likely to fall short on without care are iron and B vitamins (rich in red meat), selenium (fish and offal) and zinc (offal and meat).

Many vegetarian slimmers also cut down on, or out, dairy products such as cheese, and eggs – partly because they can be high in calories and fat and sometimes because not all vegetarians eat dairy or eggs anyway. This may mean a possible shortfall in calcium and/or protein. (Eggs are also a good source of iron.)

What you need to do to replace the nutrients from meat, poultry and fish is to eat plenty of dark leafy green vegetables and salads, pulses, wholegrains, nuts and seeds, dried peaches and apricots (for iron, selenium and B vitamins). If you don't eat dairy, good sources of vegan calcium are poppy seeds, sesame seeds, tofu, fortified soya milk, almonds, soya beans, figs, haricot beans, spinach, brazil nuts, chickpeas, kale, white bread, broccoli, spring greens and white cabbage.

Good sources of vegan protein are tofu, Quorn, pulses, textured vegetable protein (TVP), nuts, soya milk, pasta and wholegrains.

If you do eat dairy produce, go for low-fat types such as skimmed milk, yoghurt and cottage cheese most of the time, which will still provide you with calcium and protein, and save medium- or higher-fat varieties, such as Cheddar cheese, for less frequent use (or in much smaller quantities). In fact, by avoiding fish you may be low on the essential fatty acids in the omega-6 group. Replace these with flaxseeds, walnuts, rapeseed oil and groundnut oil, or take an omega-3 supplement (1,000mg a day).

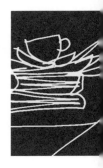

If you follow these guidelines and try to get as varied a diet as possible, you shouldn't fall short of any nutrients.

If you are thinking of following a vegetarian regime just to lose weight, do bear in mind that there are good and bad vegetarian diets, and high-calorie and low-calorie vegetarian diets. Although, statistically, vegetarians are, on average, slimmer than non-vegetarians, there is no cast-iron guarantee that you will, indeed, lose weight by giving up animal foods. I have known vegetarians become overweight on a diet of pastries, cheese pies, oily pasta, sugary desserts and chocolate. It is surprising how many vegetarians do have a sweet tooth.

you and your life

237

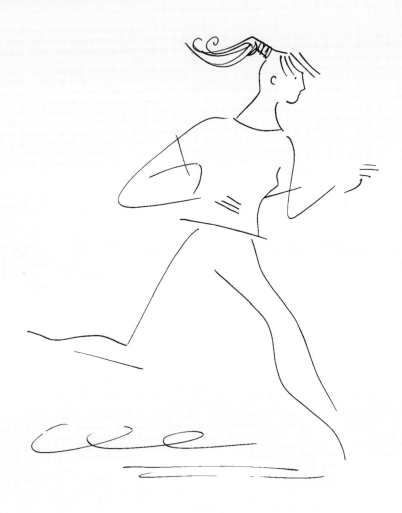

It is said most people dieting to lose weight do so for vanity rather than health. It should be the other way round, as obesity is one of the major causes of – or contributing factors to – a long list of health problems, with over 30,000 people dying each year from obesity-related illness. Yet even small losses in weight by obese people can result in a better health profile.

Many overweight people are also unfit – as fatness doesn't predispose to exercise – which is another negative health factor. As you'll discover throughout this book, regular exercise is a vital part of both weight maintenance and weight loss. Exercise is also vital for good health: hundreds of studies have concluded that regular activity protects against many diseases and increases lifespan – so people who exercise are slimmer, healthier and live longer. In this section, the questions look at all the many aspects of how your weight and fitness affect your health.

you and your health and fitness

Q177

What are the main links between weight and health?

An average body weight (BMI 20–25) is associated with your highest chance of good health. Overweight can affect health in various ways, severe obesity causing a reduction in lifespan of up to 20 years. Question 22 has already described links between overweight and health. Here are a few more facts and figures:

• Each year around 10,000 people in the UK and 70,000 in Europe develop cancer because they're fat. In 2004, Cancer Research UK reported that keeping to a healthy weight could save an estimated 6,800 women a year and 4,000 men from the disease.

• The cancers most affected by body weight are uterine (womb) cancer, breast cancer, kidney cancer and cancers of the bowel and oesophagus, while there is a link between prostate cancer in men and overweight. Excess body fat is metabolically active tissue, which produces cancer-causing hormones.

• The link between type-2 (non-insulin-dependent) diabetes (NIDD) and overweight is very strong. For example obese women aged 30–55 have 40 times greater risk of developing the disease than those with a BMI less than 22.

• Middle-aged adults who have diabetes and/or high blood pressure (a high proportion of whom will also be overweight) are more likely to suffer from dementia.

• Obesity increases the risk of developing high blood pressure and its incidence in overweight adults is nearly three times higher than in non-overweight adults. High blood pressure is a risk factor for heart disease.

• Even at body weights only 10% above average, deaths from coronary heart disease are increased. It's now thought that obesity is an independent risk factor, as well as increasing incidence of other risk factors for CHD, including high blood pressure, raised cholesterol, abdominal fat and insulin resistance.

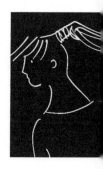

• Swedish research found that women who have been obese for long periods have brain atrophy directly linked to their weight – for every extra BMI point at age 70 the risk of Alzheimer's increased by 36 percent.

• Intra-abdominal fat (central fat distribution) is a particular risk factor for a variety of conditions and premature death. For example, in some studies it has been even more closely linked with NIDD than overall overweight, and it is closely linked with insulin resistance. People with excess abdominal fat have a higher risk of coronary heart disease and high blood pressure than those with fat on hips and thighs. IAF is also associated with increased risk of hormonal cancers, especially breast cancer, ovulatory dysfunction and sleep apnoea.

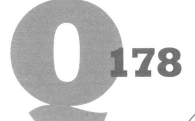

Q178

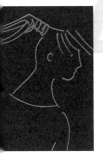

For most, keeping a BMI around 20–25 offers the greatest protection against weight-related disorders. Health risks due to increased weight rise gradually almost in line with the weight you put on, rather than how long you've been at a particular weight, though the longer you've been overweight the more likely it may be that you'll have weight-related problems, even if you keep your (over)weight stable.

Obviously, if you put on a stone or two for a few months and then lose it, you are unlikely to suffer health problems related to that. Or, if you've always been slim and only in the last few weeks put on half a stone or so, again it is unlikely that any weight-related health problems will result. Check out your BMI (see Question 26) to see what your risk of health problems is, before considering losing weight.

In fact, if you repeatedly put on weight and then lose it (the 'yo-yo syndrome'), that also increases risk of health problems, so many experts believe it's better to maintain a slightly high stable weight than to keep 'yo-yoing'.

you and your health and fitness

242

Q179

How overweight do you have to be before you get health problems?

The general consensus is that once BMI reaches about 27–8, risk of getting ill health begins to increase considerably and over 30 you're officially classed as obese. Question 26 shows you the different bands of BMI and what each means.

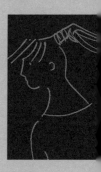

However, different professionals with different specialities disagree on what exactly an ideal weight is, and the starting point for weight-related problems. For instance, one report in the *European Heart Journal* concluded that, for middle-aged women, the healthiest BMI to have the least chance of metabolic risk factors for coronary heart disease is 22 or less, and another report found women who gained only 20lb (9kg) from their teens to middle age doubled their risk of heart attack. And yet for prevention of osteoporosis and, indeed, to avoid the yo-yo dieting syndrome, many experts believe for middle-aged women a BMI of 22 is too low.

A good indicator of health risk is having a large waist measurement, with or without a high BMI. For more on that, see Questions 47, 196 and elsewhere.

Q180 Does being overweight shorten lifespan?

We know obesity is linked with a wide range of health problems (see Questions 22 and 177), and, as some of these are life threatening, then obesity can be indirectly responsible for shortening life for people who develop these illnesses. We do also have some concrete evidence of exactly how obesity can shorten lifespan.

For instance, one US study of over 300,000 people found obesity increases risk of death from natural causes for a man aged between 40 and 50 to that of a male nearly 6 years older, and risk for a similarly aged woman increased to that of a woman 6.4 years older. A further study, this time using over 1 million US adults, also supported an increase in risk of death from all causes, including cardiovascular disease and cancer, throughout the range of moderate to severe overweight for both men and women in all age groups.

The consensus worldwide seems to be that risk of premature death increases on a reasonably level curve upwards once BMI goes over 25, with a much steeper curve after 30. At moderately high BMIs, abdominal obesity (central fat distribution) is an additional factor (see Question 196) – i.e. if you have much of your surplus fat around your middle even though your BMI is only moderately high (say 26–29), risk of early death is increased.

Problems are also increased if you have other risk factors for premature death as well as obesity – for instance, high blood pressure, high cholesterol, and/or you smoke or have diabetes. If you also take no exercise, then that too may increase risk of shortened lifespan.

HOWEVER! There is always some research that will come out and seem to prove the opposite to the bulk of evidence. A US study of 22,000 men has discovered that it is fitness not fatness that matters when it comes to prolonging life. They say that unfit, lean men are more likely to die young than fit, fat ones. Another US study actually concluded that those who are just a little overweight have a lower risk of death than those of normal weight or too thin. And yet another 2005 study from Finland concluded that people who diet die slightly younger than people who stay fat.

Perhaps my best advice is to stay a reasonable weight, eat a healthy diet and take plenty of regular exercise for a long and healthy life.

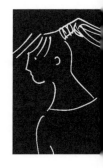

you and your health and fitness

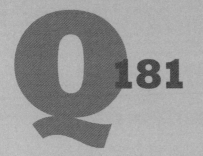

Q181

I am overweight but I feel perfectly healthy, so why should I worry?

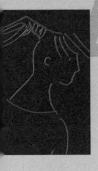

Many overweight people are currently quite healthy. If you're young, you're especially likely not to be showing visible signs of ill health. Were your arteries to be examined, though, they might well show fatty deposits, or a check-up might reveal problems (e.g. raised cholesterol, high blood pressure, insulin resistance, etc.).

There's also undoubtedly a percentage of overweight people who reach old age with hardly a day's illness – figures I quote are averages, and some people are bound to be the lucky ones who aren't average, but please don't forget that a BMI over 30 (about 20% overweight) IS a predictor of ill health later in life. So, if you are young, don't think you'll necessarily 'get away with it' forever.

You do, though, reduce chances of ill health due to obesity if you've no other negative symptoms or risk factors. So, if you don't smoke, take plenty of exercise, have normal blood pressure and blood cholesterol, your surplus weight is evenly distributed rather than mostly around your middle, your close family are all healthy, then your chances of staying healthy are much higher.

Q 182

If I've been fat for a long time, can I reverse ill health if I lose weight, and how much do I need to lose?

A It's never too late. Studies show that, in a 16 stone person, a 10% weight reduction affords significant improvement in health, and may reduce premature mortality by 25%. The Royal College of Physicians says that, with a 10% weight loss, blood pressure and cholesterol reduce and diabetes is less likely or better controlled. If very overweight, you'd probably notice improvements with smaller losses – for example, blood pressure begins reducing almost as soon as you begin losing weight.

An ideal weight range is a BMI of 20–25, but better to lose at least SOME weight than not even try because you think you'd never get near this. Weight loss for health is relative – someone with a BMI of 35 reduces risk of ill health and premature death by lowering their BMI to 29; someone with a BMI of 29 reduces the risk by getting down to 25. The slimmer you get, down to a reasonable BMI, the greater your chances of a long healthy life. However, professionals do find that people have more chance of maintaining weight loss if they aim for small losses, and it's the maintenance that's important.

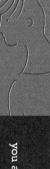

you and your health and fitness

Q183

What's the healthiest slimming diet in the world?

In general terms, a healthy slimming diet is one that's similar to a normal healthy eating diet – high in natural foods, such as fruit, vegetables, wholegrains and pulses, and with sufficient protein and a little fat – but with the calories it contains reduced to a sufficiently low level to produce slow to steady weight loss. A basic healthy diet is explained in detail in Chapter 2 and in particular in Questions 63–83. For many people, a calorie reduction of about 500 a day will be sufficient to produce the desired weight loss and, again, for many people, the best way to reduce the calorie content of a basic healthy diet is to reduce portion sizes slightly, particularly of the high-density, high-fat foods.

One of the great advantages of slimming on a really healthy type of diet is that, as you lose weight, you also reduce your risk of various modern Western diseases associated with poor diet. For example, up to 80% of bowel and breast cancer may be preventable through diet changes, and scientists have found that women who follow a healthy diet cut their risk of dying from heart disease by 30%. Problems such as diverticulitis, constipation, fatigue and dry skin – to name but a few – can also be helped with good diet.

As for the healthiest slimming diet in the world, perhaps there isn't really such a thing. For one, we have so many different foods to choose from, not only in this country, but from country to country. The choices vary so much that THE perfect healthy slimming diet would be very hard to define in terms of which actual foods should be eaten, in what quantities. All I can do is show you examples of what 'a' healthy diet looks like, rather than 'the' healthy diet – and leave the fine-tuning of the diet up to you. People do also vary in their nutritional needs, according to a variety of factors – their current health, age, activity levels, etc. So pinpointing a perfect diet for everyone is not possible.

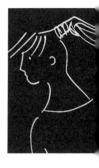

Unless you have a particular health problem, though, I wouldn't worry too much about the 'fine-tuning' aspect of your slimming programme. If you bear the general healthy-eating principles in mind – particularly with regard to choosing whole natural foods low on the Glycaemic Index (see Question 66) and keeping a watch on your total fat, saturates and trans fat intake and your sugar intake – and also watch portion size and between-meal snacking, you should do well. You could also get your doctor to refer you to a dietitian for personal help.

you and your health and fitness

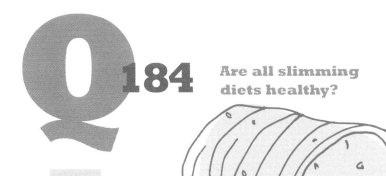

Q184

Are all slimming diets healthy?

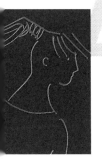

No. Typical examples of potentially unhealthy diets are any that reduce calories too low for optimum nutrient intake and may also cause problems like low blood sugar – i.e. 'crash' diets. Others are diets that limit the types of food you can eat, so you may suffer nutrient deficiencies.

There's evidence that high-protein, low-carb diets may be unhealthy, as can vegetarian diets if a suitably wide range of foods isn't eaten. High-fat, low-carb diets are generally unhealthy and even calorie-counting can problematic if you aren't sensible – you might lose weight on 1,250 calories a day of chocolate, but it's not healthy.

The US Department of Agriculture produced a report on a number of popular dieting methods and came out in favour of low-fat, high-carb as the best and healthiest way to slim. The World Health Organization endorses this.

Question 84 lists the top 6 popular diets, giving each my star rating. Go for those that did well and you'll know you have a healthy diet. However, I'd always advise you to visit your doctor and get referred to a dietitian, especially if you have health problems.

Q185

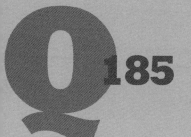

Are all healthy diets slimming?

There's more potential to lose weight on a healthy diet, mainly because it is harder to eat too many calories on a diet containing the recommended amounts of fruits, vegetables, salads, complex carbs, lean protein, etc. A healthy diet is high in 'bulk' but fairly low on density (calories per gram weight). However, if you don't pay attention to portion size or you snack on hefty amounts of healthy nuts or bread between meals, you could easily exceed required calories and put on weight.

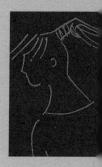

The only way to lose weight is to create an energy deficit (see Question 15) – by burning more calories than you take in. There is some small advantage to be gained by the type of food you eat (e.g. protein and carbs tend to store fewer calories on you than fat does), but in the total scheme of things the difference won't be huge.

There are many other advantages to eating a healthy diet – for example, you are less likely to suffer from hunger pangs. And, of course, you'll be doing your body more good by slimming on a healthy diet, as Question 183 explains.

Q186

Are there any healthy fats that can help you lose weight?

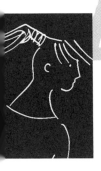

Fats are discussed in detail in Questions 71 and 72, so go back and read them. There is a type of fat called CLA, found in meat and dairy produce, which trials have shown to effect increased weight loss over a period of weeks. You do, however, need to eat vast quantities of these products in order to get enough CLA, so that blows that one (although supplements are available).

An adequate intake of the essential fatty acid omega-3 group may also help weight loss, and certainly, these healthy fats are in shortfall in many of our diets, and so getting extra of them will be of benefit to many people, even if weight loss doesn't result. These oils are found in oily fish, flaxseeds, hemp oil, pumpkin seeds and various plant oils (again see Questions 71 and 72 for more detail).

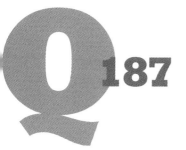

Q187

If crash dieting isn't healthy, why has his doctor put my very overweight husband on a very-low-calorie liquid diet?

Obese people with life-threatening conditions (or sometimes before an operation) may be put on a monitored very-low-calorie diet (VLCD) to get their weight down and thus reduce the risk of early death or problems during anaesthesia or surgery. It is often a 'last resort', when attempts to get the patient to lose weight on a normal calorie-controlled diet have failed.

Obesity specialists recognize this as a valid and useful way to slim patients, and the World Health Organization says VLCDs should be reserved for rapid weight loss on medical grounds in patients with a BMI over 30. I assume your husband meets these requirements, hence the treatment. VLCDs aren't recommended otherwise.

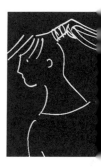

you and your health and fitness

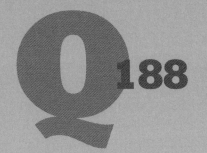

Q188

Is yo-yo dieting bad for me, and can I lose weight after years of yo-yoing?

More common among women, yo-yo dieting (or 'weight cycling') involves periods of very low calorie intake and weight loss followed by the weight returning and perhaps more gained. Women whose weight fluctuates constantly are at greater risk of various health problems than those maintaining a permanently raised weight.

One study found yo-yo dieting raised risk of heart disease in women. A mere three cycles of losing and regaining as little as 10 pounds appears to increase risk by 12%. This seems to be because yo-yoing reduces levels of 'good' HDL cholesterol in the blood. Research also found long-term immune function decreases in proportion to the number of yo-yo cycles. Loss of more than 10 pounds on 5 occasions or more made an immune system one-third less efficient.

There are also possible links with high blood pressure, diabetes and gallstones, and it can also result in deficiencies of nutrients like calcium or omega-3s, possibly resulting in higher risk of diseases like osteoporosis. Yo-yoing may also be bad psychologically, producing long-term feelings of frustration, depression, failure and low self-esteem.

The good news is that it's never too late to repair at least some of the damage. Maintain a reasonable body weight, eat a healthy balanced diet and take regular exercise, and you can improve general health, blood fat and cholesterol profile and bone density.

As to whether you can lose weight after years of yo-yoing, the idea that it permanently lowers metabolic rate isn't altogether true. If you lose weight and then regain it, there's a tendency for your body to contain less lean tissue (muscle) than before. This is because you lose lean tissue as well as fat, but when most people put weight back on they regain mostly fat and little lean tissue. Fat is less metabolically active than lean tissue, so you're then predisposed to having a lower metabolic rate, making it harder to lose weight next time.

However, most studies indicate lean tissue change isn't great – particularly if you haven't crash-dieted – nor is metabolic rate reduction. Even if you've less lean tissue than you'd have had if you'd never dieted, it's possible to increase that and metabolic rate again through exercise.

You also need to make certain lifestyle and attitude changes to help yourself lose weight sensibly and keep it off. Be happy with a final weight that isn't too low. For previous yo-yo dieters, a BMI of around 25 is a better goal than a lower one. Aiming too low is a typical cause of the start of the yo-yo cycle. Aim for slow, steady weight loss and recognize that as you near your target weight, weight loss will slow down.

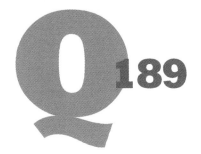

'Low blood sugar' or hypoglycaemia can arise for various reasons. Symptoms include feeling dizzy/weak, palpitations, hand tremor, lethargy/fatigue, irritability, feeling 'spaced out' and perhaps hungry. Blood sugar levels are influenced mainly by food intake – when you eat levels rise – and by insulin released by the pancreas to convert sugar to fuel or store it as fat. Once this is done, blood sugar levels should be normal, but this isn't always the case. Potentially serious hypoglycaemia can occur in diabetes when food intake doesn't match insulin levels and is relieved by immediate intake of sugary food.

In non-diabetics, hypoglycaemia can occur frequently or occasionally, mildly or more strongly, depending on the individual, their diet and circumstances. The reasons it may happen when slimming include:

• Lengthy fasting: if following inadvisable diets in which you go many hours without eating, low blood sugar is likely. A suitable snack or meal will restore it.

• Not enough to eat: periods of surviving on very-low-calorie meals, even if regular, may induce low blood

sugar simply because the energy in what you eat is absorbed too quickly. It's important not to diet on too few calories (see Question 85) and also to eat the right foods.
• Bingeing on sugary foods: it's common for dieters to get a physical/psychological urge for something sweet. This may be more apparent in women before a period, or when people are under stress and extra stress hormones are produced, as hormones can affect insulin production and blood sugar levels.
• Hard exercise: if you're not only dieting but having long periods of exercise, you may suffer low blood sugar because your body will be using sugar for energy. If doing more exercise than usual, you need to eat properly and/or have a small complex-carb, low-GI (see Question 66) snack beforehand.

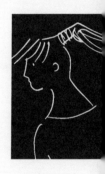

The answer to avoiding these situations is eating properly. Apart from having regular meals and small between-meal snacks, avoiding simple carbs (particularly sweets, biscuits, cakes and sugary drinks) and ensuring you get plenty of low-GI foods, also:
• Avoid caffeine (it can cause release of extra insulin, making low blood sugar worse).
• Avoid smoking as this, too, disrupts the body's regulation of blood sugars.
• Eat adequate amounts of chromium-rich foods, like broccoli, shellfish, wheatgerm, nuts, fruits and veg, as chromium is an important factor in blood sugar regulation.
• Regularly eat oily fish, flaxseeds and other sources of omega-3s. Research shows they may help regulate blood sugar by increasing insulin sensitivity.

you and your health and fitness

257

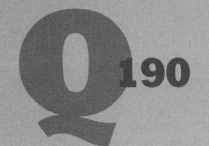

Q190 Can you recommend a good slimming diet for a diabetic?

Diabetes UK says it doesn't provide a special diet for diabetics, as the diet they should follow is similar to the kind of healthy diet appropriate for most people. It is important for diabetics to try to control their weight, or lose weight if necessary. Type-2 diabetes may be improved or even cured via weight loss.

However, it's worth mentioning a few extra nutritional facts that may help if you're diabetic and trying to lose weight:

• Eating 'little and often' really IS the way to go for you, to help keep blood sugar levels even. Don't go more than $2\frac{1}{2}$ hours without something to eat during waking hours.

• Be extra sure to get plenty of foods with a low Glycaemic Index into your diet (see Question 66). These will also help stabilize your blood sugars and help keep hunger at bay.

• Don't try dieting on a plan very low in fat. A little fat with your meals helps the meal take longer to be absorbed and, again, will help maintain even blood sugar levels. The same applies to protein. So, at every meal, aim to get some low-GI carb, some fat and some protein.

• Diabetics may have kidney problems, so drink enough water to help them work well (but not too much, which can overtax the kidneys – about 6 glasses of water a day will be good in normal circumstances).

• Diabetics may be more prone to infections, so get plenty of fresh fruits, salads and vegetables in your diet for the antioxidant carotenes and vitamin C, which help to protect you. Get the antioxidant zinc from foods such as nuts, seeds and lean red meat, and get vitamin E, another antioxidant important for diabetics, from nuts, seeds and plant oils.

• Research shows that a diet rich in oily fish, nuts, seeds and plant oils may help to regulate the blood sugar levels.

• Don't be tempted to try dieting too quickly – aim for a weekly weight loss of no more than half a pound (225g) (after the first week of slimming), which should be possible by reducing your daily calorie intake by only 250 or so. If you try to reduce your calories down too low, you may create problems in maintaining even blood sugar levels.

Diabetics should always discuss diet with their doctor and not follow any new diet without their knowledge.

Diabetes UK (formerly the British Diabetic Association), 10 Queen Anne Street, London W1G 9LH tel 0207 424 1000 www.diabetes.org.uk

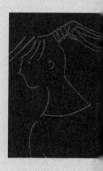

you and your health and fitness

Q191 What are the health advantages of a detox diet?

Sometimes there are few advantages, if any, as many of the 'detox' regimes that are offered in the newspapers and magazines are of little benefit to most people. A detox is supposed to rid your body of all the pollutants that you, or your environment, have been putting into it – e.g. 'bad' foods containing additives, preservatives or too much fat, pesticides, herbicides, hormones, heavy metals, smoke and air pollution, alcohol, tobacco, medicines... and more.

The idea with most detoxes is that you eat or drink natural – and naturally detoxing – items and avoid everything likely to add to your body's pollution levels. Some detoxes are little more than fasts, and others ask you to spend a lot of money on bottled potions, pills and so on, which really isn't necessary.

The British Dietetic Association says that 'detox' is a meaningless word, and toxicology experts at the University of California said in 2005 that there is no scientific evidence that 'detox' diets help to remove toxins from the body and that detox regimes which

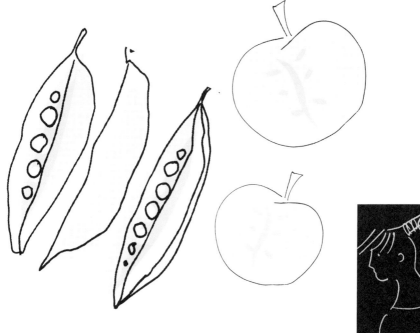

amount to 'protracted starvation' may, ironically, slow down the metabolic rate and the breakdown of fat stores. They conclude that strict detox diets may pose a significant health risk.

My opinion? A gentle 'detox' high in fruit, vegetables, wholegrains and omega-3 oils may, for some, be a good kick-start to a slimming diet, because it will reduce your calorie intake significantly and help reduce fluid bloating, but don't stay on any detox regime for long periods. I would also not advise people prone to yo-yo dieting, low blood sugar or eating disorders to follow a strict detox regime.

you and your health and fitness

Q192

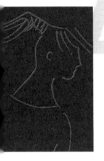

All detoxes I've come across reduce calorie intake significantly and would thus almost certainly help you lose weight – but NOT because toxins have been keeping you fat. Much of the weight loss will be fluid. Detoxes tend to be very low on carbohydrate, which helps retain water. A low-carb diet therefore encourages water elimination and in a week you might lose several pounds of fluid as well as a pound or two of fat.

I wouldn't recommend a detox regime for long periods as they're too low in calories, so they're not much use for long-term weight loss, unless on a 'one week on detox, three weeks of normal healthy eating' basis. I'd also not advise people prone to yo-yo dieting to follow a detox, nor people prone to low blood sugar. A detox is a crash diet by any other name, and ordinary gentle calorie reduction is best for both these groups.

For many, however, a good detox gets them into the right frame of mind for healthier eating and weight loss. In other words, it can be a very good start.

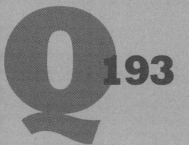

Q193 What's the best slimming diet for someone with high blood pressure?

If you're overweight and have high blood pressure you can almost immediately reduce it by losing weight. Follow guidelines for a good healthy slimming diet, but also bear the following in mind:

• Lose weight steadily. Research shows yo-yo dieting can make high blood pressure worse.

• Limit salt intake to no more than 4g daily – about a level teaspoon, equivalent to 1.8g of actual sodium. Don't forget that salt occurs in many ready-made products, so cut right back on these. For more on salt, see Question 133. There are salt substitutes such as LoSalt.

• Eat plenty of potassium-rich foods, as a high potassium intake can help lower blood pressure. These include most fruits and veg, dried apricots, nuts and pulses.

• Other nutrients that may lower blood pressure include calcium (low-fat dairy produce, dark leafy greens), magnesium (nuts, seeds, wholegrains, green vegetables), omega-3 fats (oily fish, flaxseeds).

• Garlic and soluble fibre (found in fruits, pulses and vegetables) may also help.

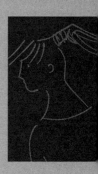

Q194

What's the best slimming diet for someone with arthritis?

There are two types of arthritis: osteoarthritis and rheumatoid arthritis. The first is a degenerative condition of the joints that often occurs with age, giving stiffness and pain in the affected joints. Overweight can make the problems worse, as the joints have to bear a greater load.

Sufferers should follow a basic healthy slimming diet (see Questions 183–5) containing reasonably high amounts of antioxidant vitamins C and E, which have been found in some trials to help osteoarthritis. Cod liver oil and other fish oils may also help.

Rheumatoid arthritis is a chronic inflammatory condition involving multiple joints, when the immune system appears to overreact to some stimulant. Joints may swell and there may be pain. The causes aren't fully understood. Various foods have been cited as making it worse, but the list of foods which may affect some people (but not others) is long. These include all members of the 'nightshade family' (potatoes, tomatoes, aubergines and peppers), all foods high in saturated fat, coffee, alcohol, citrus fruits, all dairy produce, wheat, corn, and nuts.

If you feel any of these do seem to aggravate your arthritis, replace them with similar foods. For example, rice instead of potatoes, water and herb tea instead of coffee and alcohol, soya products instead of dairy, and rye bread or rice crackers instead of wheat and corn products. Instead of nuts you could try seeds, or a little extra of good-quality plant and fish oils in your diet.

If unsure which foods may make your arthritis worse, you could go through the list, eliminating one food at a time to see if symptoms improve. However, elimination diets are best undertaken with the help of a trained dietitian. The problem with trying to diagnose a food intolerance is that rheumatoid arthritis tends to go through periods of remission, so it's hard to be sure whether an improvement may be due to a removed food, or because coincidentally you have entered a remission.

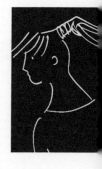

Foods that may help the symptoms of rheumatoid arthritis are oily fish, which contain the essential fats omega-3s, and fruit and veg, again probably because of their antioxidants. People with rheumatoid arthritis show low levels of the mineral selenium, so a diet with adequate selenium could help too – find it in nuts, seeds, lentils, fish, pork and wholegrains. In other trials, the spice turmeric has been found to help – add it to curries, stews, etc. – and some people say evening primrose oil helps.

Lastly, a completely vegetarian or vegan diet has been found to help prevent rheumatoid arthritis in some people or minimize symptoms. As a compromise, you could take fish-oil supplements while you do this or, if you prefer, try flaxseed oil, which is also omega-3 rich.

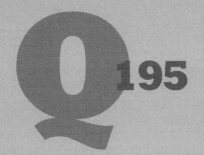

Q195

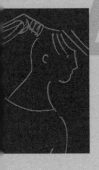

The apple shape (fat mainly around abdomen and waist – also called central fat distribution) is linked with health problems like coronary heart disease and diabetes, whereas pear shape (heavy hips, bottom and thighs) doesn't appear to present the same level of risk.

This shape is predominantly a male phenomenon, although women are more prone to develop apple shape in midlife, particularly after menopause as female hormones are present in smaller amounts so the shape tends to become more 'male'. There's also evidence that abdominal fat develops when under long-term stress. The hormone cortisol is released during stress, and it seems high levels encourage central fat accumulation. Research at Yale University studied 60 women and found the more stress they were under, the more fat they stored around their stomachs. So those most likely to develop this shape are stressed men of any age, and older stressed women.

The apple effect can be minimized with a sensible diet, regular exercise and stress-reduction techniques (exercise is a good stress-buster). See also Questions 26, 46 and 47.

Q196

Why does overweight increase your risk of heart disease?

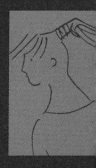

A Until recently, the consensus was that overweight increases risk of heart disease (or coronary arterial disease), as well as other cardiovascular diseases (CVDs), including stroke, as it predisposes to other cardiovascular risk factors, including high blood pressure, raised cholesterol and impaired glucose tolerance and diabetes.

However, long-term studies now show obesity is an 'independent' risk factor – meaning that, even if you had none of the health problems above, it could still increase your risk of CVD. These studies link weight gain with the risk of developing CHD, and the fatter you are the greater the risk. Also, intra-abdominal fat is more closely linked with CVD than any other body fat distribution. Evidence is so strong that the American Heart Association has listed obesity as one of the primary risk factors for CHD.

If you already have heart disease and are overweight, it's important to try to reduce your weight to within 10% of a normal range (i.e. a BMI of around 27–28), as excess weight increases the load on your heart, especially during exercise, which is generally encouraged for heart patients.

you and your health and fitness

267

Q197 What is the ideal weight and diet for a healthy heart?

Most research shows people with the healthiest hearts are quite thin. The World Health Organization says death from heart disease is increased in individuals only 10% above average weight, while recent research suggested that, for middle-aged women, a healthy BMI is only 22 – less than most experts would cite as healthy for the prevention of osteoporosis. Looking at prevention of premature death from all causes, however, the consensus is that BMI has to get well over 26 before chances increase significantly. So, the ideal weight for heart health is hotly debated.

Again 'central fat distribution' is a factor – if you're apple-shaped, but within a normal range BMI, risk of heart disease increases. If at the heavier end of normal-range BMI (i.e. around 25), but not an apple shape, you probably don't have increased risk. If young, though, I suggest you try to maintain your BMI around 22 for women and 23 for men, especially if there's a family history of heart disease or stroke.

An ideal diet for a healthy heart is one that doesn't put on too much weight. If you need to lose weight, ensure your diet includes plenty of foods thought to help your heart in other ways:

• Oily fish and fish oils – the special omega-3s (DHA and EPA) fish contain is good at preventing blood clots, lowering blood fat levels and helping reduce blood pressure. Interestingly, much research shows that the kind of diet recommended to help prevent or manage heart disease – very low in fat and high in carbs – although reducing 'bad' LDL blood cholesterol, actually tends to increase harmful triglycerides. If, though, you regularly eat oily fish (or take supplements) and take regular exercise, trigylceride levels tend not to increase.

• Antioxidant-rich fruit and vegetables. Vitamins A, C and E and the minerals zinc and selenium help protect your heart by combating free radicals. Find vitamin beta-carotene (becomes vitamin A in the body) in orange, red, yellow and dark-green fruits and vegetables; find vitamin C in most fruits and vegetables; and find vitamin E in plant oils, nuts, seeds, dark greens, avocados and sweet potatoes. Nuts, seeds and fish contain selenium and zinc, while red meat is also a good source of zinc. Tea and red wine also contain beneficial antioxidants, but wine should be limited to one or two glasses a day.

• Flavonoids. These special 'phytochemicals' can help your heart – find them in citrus fruits, blackcurrants, melon, berry fruits and red peppers.

• B vitamins including folate – find them in liver, wholegrains, pulses and leafy vegetables.

• Soluble fibre – find this in oats, pulses and many fruits and vegetables.

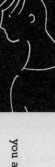

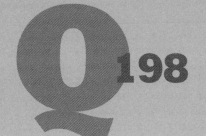

Q 198 Should I go to the doctor for help with losing weight?

Doctors won't thank me for advising everyone who needs to lose weight to go to the surgery for advice – they would be overrun and unable to cope, as up to two-thirds of us are overweight! I think you need to use common sense to decide whether a visit to the doctor is wise. Here are some occasions when it may be so:

• If you've been putting on weight and feel that you haven't altered your eating or exercise patterns. If you have other symptoms (e.g. tiredness, lethargy, coldness), you should certainly go. Unexplained weight gain may be a sign of an underlying health problem.

• If you're very overweight – with a body mass index over 30 – you should get a thorough check-up and the doctor will probably want to give you advice on lifestyle changes you could make – diet, exercise and so on. He/she may refer you to a dietitian and even give you a prescription for visits to your local gym – in the UK, a standard prescription charge allows you a monitored course of exercise at the leisure centre, gym or swimming pool in participating areas.

Obese people are at increased risk of all kinds of health problems, which is why it is important to involve your doctor. Many obese people have tried to lose weight themselves and find it too difficult, so seeing the doctor may help you to lose the weight this time.

• If you think you may have an eating disorder, it is a good idea to see your doctor, who may refer you to a specialist for help.

• If you are pregnant or thinking of becoming pregnant and are overweight, you should see your doctor.

• If you have repeatedly tried to lose weight and failed. Your doctor may be able to give you advice – or may even suggest a slimming pill.

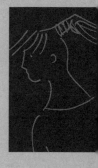

Some doctors are not as sympathetic as they should be with overweight people – such unsympathetic doctors should realize that a few minutes' helpful consultation with an overweight person now may save much NHS money (half a billion pounds a year of it) and much of their time in future years. Also, in my experience, some doctors don't know a great deal about sensible slimming or nutrition, although some, of course, do. Which side yours falls into is a bit of a lottery. If you feel you aren't getting good advice, ask to be referred to the community dietitian.

So when is it NOT necessary to visit your doctor about a surplus weight problem? I'd say if you are in good health otherwise and have decided that you need to shed a stone or so, then you may follow a good healthy slimming plan, or you may like to join a slimming club for support and advice.

Q199 Can you be overweight and yet fit?

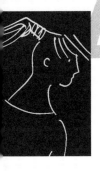

You can achieve both cardiovascular and muscle fitness while carrying too much body fat (see Question 27). Some rugby players, say – are fit while clinically overweight. As you get older it becomes less likely, if very overweight, that you'll be fit, as the more obese you are, the less exercise you do, and it's exercise that keeps you fit.

The other point is that certain people with excellent muscular strength, if not excellent CV health – for example, body builders – may be overweight according to BMI (see Question 26) but not according to body-fat percentage. However, they may not be 'all-round' fit – their heart-lung fitness might not be top-notch and their suppleness poor. True fitness is not just being aerobically fit, but also fit in terms of strength and flexibility, etc.

So, although you may have a satisfactory level of fitness, if you're carrying too much body fat, you're predisposing yourself to ill health later. However, research shows that people who take regular cardiovascular exercise tend to lose weight over time, so if CV fit, you may lose weight naturally.

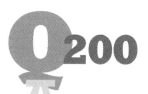

Q200   How does fitness affect weight?

If cardiovascular fit, you probably take regular aerobic exercise – a good calorie-burner, so you shouldn't have trouble keeping weight down. If you have good muscle strength, you have a high proportion of lean tissue, which is more metabolically active than fat, so you burn more calories even when inactive. This also helps keep body fat down. However, as muscle weighs more than fat, some find that after long-term healthy eating and exercise including weight training, they lose fat but don't weigh less.

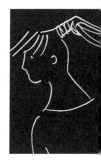

Q201   In what ways does being fit affect health?

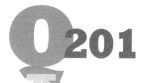

It's generally held that if you're physically fit then you're better able to ward off illness because your immune system is fitter. Numerous studies conclude that you're also at less risk of contracting cardiovascular disease and some cancers, arthritis and other health problems. Also some forms of exercise can lower blood pressure. If you exercise to keep weight down, you'll also be less at risk from the health problems that affect overweight people.

you and your health and fitness

273

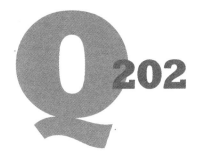

Q202 How does exercise help with weight control when it increases appetite?

Exercise doesn't automatically increase appetite, at least not in the short term. Indeed, there's good evidence to show that if you feel hungry after a workout, it is either lunchtime, or it is a psychological hunger rather than a physiological need. 'I've just burnt 300 calories in the gym – good, I deserve a chocolate bar!' In fact, one study came to the conclusion that people overestimate how many calories they're burning in the gym and tend to eat more calories than they have burnt to reward themselves.

There is also some evidence that you are more likely to feel the need for food after a fairly short exercise session (half an hour or so) than after a longer one – as, at least for some people, the appetite seems to be dulled by longer exercise periods. A 2005 study published in the *American Journal of Clinical Nutrition* found that, for women, vigorous short-term exercise increases appetite – especially for fatty foods – more than more moderate, longer-term exercise. A high-intensity workout meant that the women tested replaced over 90% of the calories they had just burnt off in the next meal, while low-intensity exercise caused them to replace only a third of the calories burnt.

If you do tend to feel hungry after exercise, first drink plenty of low-calorie drink, to avoid dehydration. This will help to give you a feeling of fullness, too. Then eat a small carbohydrate-rich snack such as a slice of bread or a banana, which will restore your blood sugar levels if you have been working out vigorously. After a long and vigorous session (especially if you feel dizzy or fatigued), you could take a sports energy drink.

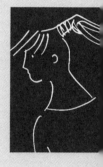

However, with sensible diet, overall your calorie intake needn't increase because of exercise. For example, a session done after breakfast means that you can use your mid-morning snack as your post-exercise energy booster, adding no extra calories to your day's intake at all. Or a late afternoon session after your mid-afternoon snack can be followed by your evening meal. Planning is all!

In general, exercise helps with weight control by burning calories – both aerobic exercise and strength (resistance) training does this. Aerobic exercise burns calories (or actual body fat) while you are doing it, and for a while afterwards, while strength training burns calories, and, by increasing your body's proportion of lean tissue, which is metabolically active, you also raise your metabolic rate long-term and burn more calories that way too. One study published in the *American Journal of Clinical Nutrition* found that weight training 3–5 times a week raises the metabolic rate by 15%.

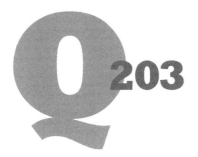

Q203

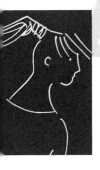

If you mean formal exercise, like gyms or organized sport, there's plenty left you can do – for example, walking is the best all-purpose exercise. All activity, even standing, uses more calories than complete inactivity, so the more active you can make your daily life, then the more calories you'll burn without having to do any 'proper' exercise. Make an effort to build extra movement into your routine. Housework can be every bit as good as a workout for calorie burning. Also think about gardening, mowing, carrying shopping, running up and down stairs, etc.

If that all sounds too boring, think of some fun ways to burn calories. How about dancing or in-line skating? Alternatively, go for some less competitive, non-team sport, like orienteering or cycling.

Don't dismiss all 'real' exercise. I know several confirmed 'exercise haters' who, when dragged along to various classes, ended up hooked and have also taken up other forms of exercise. Exercise releases hormones that make you feel better. Keep an open mind, grab a friend for moral support and give some things a try.

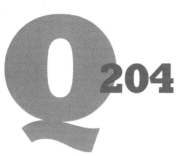

Q204 What is aerobic exercise?

Aerobic, or cardiovascular, exercise is exercise that achieves the following:
• Increases cardiac fitness, strengthening the heart and making it more efficient, thus reducing beats per minute. There is thus less strain on it during exercise and at rest.
• Increases lung capacity – increasing volume of usable air sacs as well as efficiency of oxygen exchange. If you're fit, you get more oxygen per breath and breathing rate slows.
• It burns calories and/or fat and can increase metabolic rate slightly afterwards.
• It may increase strength in muscles used (e.g. legs in running) and build a little extra lean tissue.

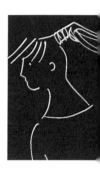

   Exercise is aerobic when it gets heart rate into the 'training zone', normally 60%–80% of maximum (see Question 222). Research shows unfit people can gain benefits in cardiovascular fitness with only short regular periods (10 minutes) of such exercise. Experts say you need to do aerobic exercise for a minimum of 3–5 times weekly, whatever your fitness. Aerobic exercise includes brisk walking, running, cycling, swimming and dancing.

you and your health and fitness

277

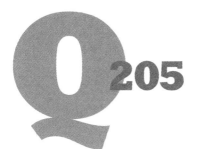

Q205 How often do I have to exercise to lose weight?

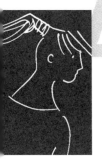

If you can lose half a pound of body fat a week through exercise, you're doing well. That would translate into seven 40-minute walking sessions at 240 calories each, which equates to the recommendation from the American College of Sports Medicine that 30 minutes or more of moderate intensity exercise, such as walking, is done on most or preferably all days of the week.

How often you need to exercise to lose weight depends on how much you want to lose, the form of exercise, and how long you exercise. For maximum weight loss, you'd have to do regular lengthy daily exercise of high aerobic intensity (e.g. running, fast cycling). If unfit, however, you need to begin any exercise programme gently and build up gradually.

Recent studies have found that regular moderate exercise achieves better results than intensive bursts and people who do a weekly intense gym session expend less energy over a week than people who regularly do moderate exercise like walking. Adding extra 'informal exercise' into daily life (see Question 203) will also help.

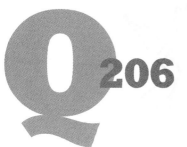

Q 206

How long do I have to exercise for at a time to lose weight?

The important factor is how long in total you exercise for over the course of, say, a week, not how long each individual session is. Much recent research shows that both short sessions and long sessions burn equal amounts of fat or calories if they add up to the same time in the end. A study at Loughborough University found that three 10-minute sessions of brisk walking a day, five days a week, achieved the same rates of calorie burn and fitness levels as five half-hour walks a week and a similar study at the University of Virginia in the USA found the same thing.

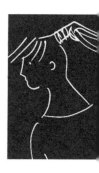

The crucial thing is that you can't go for three 10-minute walks a week and expect to burn many calories. So it's either 'short and very frequent' or 'longer and less frequent'. The choice is up to you and what fits in best with your lifestyle. Also see the answer to the previous question, which discusses the importance of the type of exercise you choose to do.

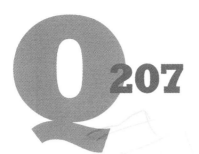

Q207

How much weight can I lose through exercise?

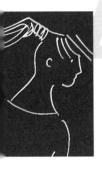

You have to work quite hard to lose more than about half a pound of body fat (225g) a week through exercise, but as long as you do exercise regularly, over and above your previous levels, then you should continue to lose weight and/or body fat down to a weight that is optimal for you, particularly if you manage to increase your muscle (lean tissue) through resistance exercise as well. When you are at or near that weight, it should then be possible to maintain a suitable weight via an exercise and diet maintenance programme.

The best combination is to exercise regularly and cut down your calorie intake slightly, to produce a weight loss of about 2lb (1kg) a week if you are very overweight, or 1lb (0.5kg) a week if you are not so overweight. Questions 205 and 206 give you more information on the duration, frequency and intensity of the exercise that you should do.

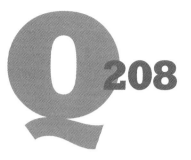

Q208

Is the best exercise for weight control 'short and sharp' or 'long and slow'?

First read Questions 204–7 to give you the background. What matters for calorie burning are the total amount of time you spend and the intensity of the exercise. As we've seen, around 4 hours a week of moderate-intensity exercise, like brisk walking, should result in weight loss over time. A similar length of time spent on a harder exercise, such as running or an advanced aerobics class, would result in more calories burnt. Alternatively, a shorter length of time spent on the harder exercise would result in the same calories burnt as the 4 hours' walking.

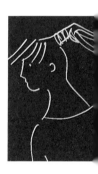

There is some evidence that short bursts of exercise are more easily fitted into people's lives and therefore they may stick with it. For some people (especially women) who find that exercise increases appetite, it may be better to do longer more moderate exercise sessions, as it seems that hard short sessions increase the appetite more.

Lastly, research shows that 30 minutes' moderate exercise (e.g. walking) a day is enough to prevent weight gain in sedentary people.

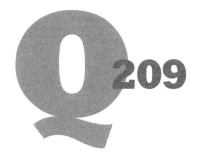

Q209

You would find that if you gave up the five-days-a-week walk and didn't alter your eating habits, you would slowly put on weight, which would prove that the walking is affecting your weight control, but not in the way you want. When we discuss how you can lose weight through exercise (see Questions 202–8), I am talking about new exercise, over and above what you have habitually been doing. You are currently exercising enough to maintain your current weight, and to lose weight you would need either to increase the amount you are doing and/or cut your calorie intake a little.

Even if you have only recently started walking your child to school, and so therefore it IS a 'new' activity, you are probably not burning up enough calories to show anything other than a very slow weight loss. If this sounds hardly believable, let me explain.

I expect your child is quite young (if he or she needs walking to school), and therefore, having done a similar thing myself for years, I know that you are probably walking to school at a leisurely pace rather than a brisk walk. In that case, you are not burning anywhere near as many calories during the daily 40 minutes as you might if you were walking alone or with an adult. You're walking 10 minutes each way, 4 times a day. A single 10-minute walk from your home to school with a child may be a distance of only about a quarter or a mile, perhaps a little more. That means you are walking perhaps a mile a day, or 5 miles a week. Research shows that you burn about 100 calories for every mile you cover (whether you walk slowly, briskly, or even run). So you are burning only about 500 calories a week in your school walks. Even if this were a 'new' exercise, it would still only produce a weekly weight loss of about one-seventh of a pound, or a pound every seven weeks.

Walking quicker on the half of the journey when you aren't with the child won't up the calories burnt – as we've seen, if you are walking a quarter of a mile, it doesn't matter what pace you go at. You need to find a longer route home and burn more calories off that way. Walking on your own, you should be able to cover about $2^1/_2$–3 miles in 40 minutes – burning nearly three times the calories of your walks with your child and burning off nearly half a pound a week. Even if extra walking isn't possible, don't get disheartened and abandon your daily walks – they will be doing your health good even if weight loss isn't apparent.

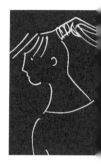

you and your health and fitness

Q210 What low-cost exercise can I do to lose weight?

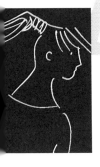

There's no need to spend a lot of money on exercise – only 16% of people in the UK belong to a gym, for instance, and most expensive exercise equipment is rarely used.

The cheapest aerobic exercise is walking, and it's also the simplest and easiest. Cycling is also quite inexpensive, although obviously you have to buy the bike. If you have a music system, you could put on some upbeat music and dance away the calories.

Simply getting more active in your everyday life can burn plenty of calories without costing you anything – you could even save money. For instance, you could walk to work instead of taking a car or bus, which would save petrol or fare. You could live without the cleaner and do housework instead of watching TV. If you have a garden, you could get out there and dig a patch to grow your own vegetables, thus saving money again.

You could also consider doing sponsored walking or cycling to raise money for charity – a great motivator.

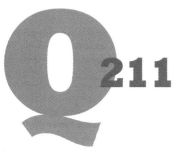

Q211 What's the best calorie-burning exercise programme for an unfit beginner?

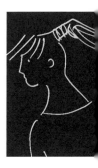

You need good regular aerobic exercise to suit your needs (see Questions 201–9). If you want to burn the maximum calories you should also begin resistance work – i.e. something to strengthen muscles and add bulk to them so metabolic rate is raised. Again, you need to start gradually and build up the resistance and number of 'reps'.

If starting at rock-bottom unfitness and if you haven't done any formal exercise before, think about getting a check-up to make sure you're in good enough health to begin, and you should always obey instructions about safe exercise. The most important thing is to go at your own pace – you're not in competition with anyone – and build up gradually. Though for most people – even elderly beginners – results are remarkably quick. You won't lose weight rapidly through exercise alone, but you'll notice a difference in your shape (particularly around the midriff at first), muscle tone and energy levels.

For more noticeable weight loss, combine your calorie-burning regime with a slightly reduced-calorie diet.

Q212

I can spare 10 minutes a day and am reasonably fit. Which exercise will burn up the most calories in that time?

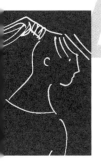

You need something you can do 'instantly'. You could skip (7 cals/minute), or step (9). Warm up and cool down by gently marching on the spot. If you fancy more expensive equipment, a rower burns about 8 cals a minute, a Stairmaster 9 and an elliptical trainer 9. Most come with a built-in calorie readout (often 'optimistic'). Even so, 10 minutes using any of these will burn around 100 calories.

Generally, exercise that works both arms and legs will burn more calories, so a rower is better than a bike, say. Also, anything done standing is harder work (e.g. a treadmill rather than a bike). Lastly, any work on an uphill incline will increase burn (e.g. a stepper or treadmill on incline). Maximize your time by 'doubling up' – for example, when you step, carry hand weights. If you increase muscle, you'll burn more calories as you exercise.

Try to make small changes in your lifestyle so you can spend a bit more time on yourself – say flexibility work three times a week. Unfit people note – these high-intensity, short-burst exercises aren't for you. You need to build up gradually.

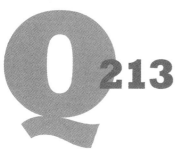

Q 213

Can you recommend any home exercise equipment to help burn calories?

There is a huge range of equipment that you can buy, from a basic skipping rope to a top-of-the-range treadmill costing thousands of pounds. The main consideration, apart from cost, is where you will keep the item(s) that you buy.

If you have to keep a folding treadmill or bike in a cupboard or an outhouse, for example, it is unlikely that you will use it. If you haven't a room to set aside where any large equipment can be left out ready to use, I'd think twice about buying anything large and settle for the rope or, at most, a rebounder, which is lightweight and set down ready to use in a second.

Bear in mind that for optimum calorie burning you need to do some strength training as well as aerobic training, so investing in a set of dumbbells or resistance bands would be a good idea.

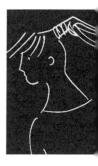

you and your health and fitness

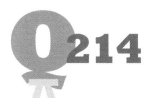

Q214

What's the best all-round programme to keep fit and slim?

You need to do regular aerobic work (see Question 204) to burn calories and keep heart and lungs fit; regular resistance training (strength work), which tones your body, keeps lean tissue (muscle) intact (or even increases it), helps boost metabolic rate and burns calories; and regular flexibility exercises to keep joints supple.

I suggest you do an aerobics programme on alternate days, and the strength work on the days you aren't doing aerobic, and that you do some stretching every day after your workout.

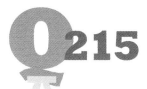

Q215

Apart from weights, which exercises build muscles?

Any aerobic exercise that works one of the major muscle groups will help to build muscle in the group worked. For example, running, cycling and step aerobics will help to build strong leg muscles. Plyometrics – jumping, bounding, hopping and leaping – have also been shown to be good for muscle building in the legs. Swimming and rowing, for example, will help to build strong arm muscles.

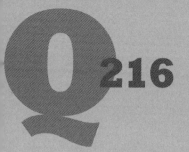

Q216

When you exercise, what is the difference between burning calories and burning fat?

When you exercise, you can use both carbohydrate (stored as glycogen in the body) and fat for fuel. In the early stages of a session, more carbs than fat are burnt (particularly with high-intensity exercise, where carbs are the body's 'preferred fuel'), but after 20 minutes the percentage of fat burnt increases. Towards the end of prolonged exercise – an hour or more – when glycogen reserves are low, fat will be supplying about 80% of your energy. The fitter you are, the better your body is at burning fat during exercise.

However, if you want to lose weight, it doesn't really matter whether you're burning body fat or using glycogen or blood sugars – you're still 'burning' calories. Any exercise you do – whether it's housework, jogging for an hour or skipping for five minutes, for example – will use calories for energy and, over time, if you create an 'energy deficit', your body will have to use its fat stores for fuel. Whether this happens while you exercise or while you sleep, you'll still 'burn' the fat and lose weight.

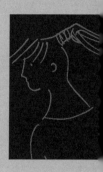

you and your health and fitness

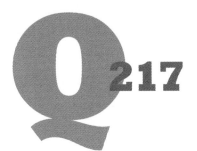

Q217

Does everybody burn calories at the same rate during exercise?

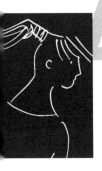

No. The less you weigh, the fewer calories you will burn, and the smaller your percentage of lean tissue (muscle), the fewer you will burn. As an example, at an average cycling pace, a 13-stone person with a high lean-tissue percentage may burn around 9 calories per minute, while an 8-stone person with a low lean-tissue percentage may burn about 5 calories per minute. This is true whatever the exercise.

Below are other examples of the difference in average calorie burning in various pursuits between first someone weighing 8 stone (51kg) and then someone weighing 13 stone (83kg).

CYCLING (10mph) 5 cals/minute and 8 cals/minute

TENNIS 5.5 cals/minute and 9 cals/minute

SWIMMING (crawl) 6.5 cals/minute and 10.5 cals/minute

RUNNING (6.5 mph) 8 cals/minute and 13 cals/minute

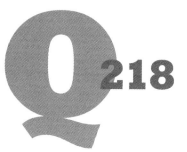

Q218

Which is the best exercise – walking, running or swimming?

It all depends on how fit you are, what you want to achieve, how much time you've got, etc. Walking is a great calorie-burning and fitness tool, particularly for beginners and the unfit, and those looking for something low-cost and easy, but does little for upper-body strength or overall flexibility.

Running burns most calories, but you can't go out and do it if unfit. You need to shower and change afterwards. Running on a hard surface may also, in time, affect weight-bearing joints and there's generally higher risk of injury. It's also no good for upper-body strength or flexibility.

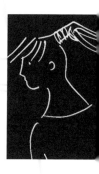

Swimming burns calories and is also a better all-round exercise for balanced body strength and flexibility – but you have to like water, be able to swim, be fairly near a pool, have the money and time, etc. Also, swimming is non-load-bearing and, therefore, not good for maintaining bone density.

So choosing the right exercise should be done with care. Think about what you want to achieve and how fit you are, and how any exercise will fit in with your life.

you and your health and fitness

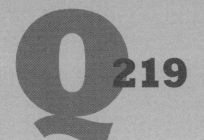

Q 219 How much exercise is too much?

It depends on your level of fitness and many other factors. In general, the less fit you are, the less exercise you can (or should) do. For example, a 20-minute walk will be plenty in one day for an unfit person, whereas a trained marathon runner will happily run several hours a day. You need to pace your activity to suit your level of fitness, and, as you get fitter, to how fit you want to be. If you use common sense and follow safety guidelines, it's unlikely you will be doing too much – what is termed 'overtraining'.

However, let's look at what 'too much' exercise is, and how it can adversely affect you. Overtraining or 'burnout' is something that may occur in athletes (usually competition-standard) when they become stale, find performance declining, feel sluggish and tired, and may have other symptoms. This is unlikely to happen to you, the beginner or moderate exerciser.

You're more likely to suffer from problems if you don't have the right technique, or try to overtax yourself slightly. You may then get aches, pains or strains, which are your body's way of telling you that you've not been going at a suitable pace for your level of fitness.

Then there are people who aren't trained athletes but become dependent on exercise – obsessional about it – and seem to spend almost every spare minute at the gym or running. This is called 'exercise addiction' and may be linked with eating disorders in some. One study in 2000 found that 18% of women studied, who were all regular exercisers, showed signs of exercise addiction.

The causes of this addiction are not certain, but one theory is that obsessional exercisers become hooked on the endorphins released when you exercise, giving the classic 'exercise high' – and withdrawal symptoms if exercise is stopped. Addicted exercisers may also be laying themselves open to a wide range of health problems. These include a reduction in the efficiency of the immune system, predisposition to osteoarthritis in the worked joints, possible cessation of periods in women, fatigue and excessive thinness.

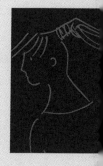

As with most aspects of life, sensible exercise is balanced and forms part of your life, rather than the major part of it. For most people, an hour a day of formal exercise would be plenty for fitness, calorie burning and health benefits, if the hour includes aerobic/strength and flexibility work and if you get other forms of activity during your normal day. People who exercise a lot should always take sufficient time to rest between sessions to allow the body to recover, and all but very experienced athletes shouldn't do high-intensity exercise for more than 90 minutes at a time to avoid suppressing the immune system.

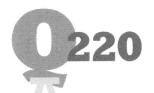

Q220 Which aerobic exercise is good for tone?

See Question 215, as 'tone' is similar to 'strength' – you get good body tone when you work muscles. Aerobic exercise can help give your body a streamlined look by burning calories and helping shed fat (a covering of fat won't allow even toned muscles to show) and also by strengthening muscles, depending upon which aerobic exercise you choose. For general toning, one of the best aerobic exercises is swimming, as it works all the muscles in the body. Up- and downhill walking are also good for the lower body, and rowing for upper-body tone. Specifically for leg muscles, choose cycling or brisk walking, including hillwork.

Q221 Apart from floor exercises, what's best for flattening bellies?

Swimming is excellent, as your abdominal muscles are used all the time. Other good exercise includes hillwalking, dancing and Ashtanga yoga. Static yoga is great, as are digging and weight training.

Q222

What are my 'training zone' and my 'maximum heart rate'?

Maximum heart rate (MHR) is the greatest number of pulse beats/minute your heart should beat. The standard way of gauging MHR is to subtract your age from 220. Your training zone is the heartbeat range at which you will gain the most benefit from aerobic exercise, and most experts give it as 60–85% of MHR, with 75% often cited as ideal – though I suggest 60% for unfit people and beginners.

EXAMPLE: You're 40. Your MHR is 180 (220–40) and training zone is 108–153 (60–85% of 180).

The aim is to keep your pulse (heart) rate at this level throughout your workout. If you go over the upper end of the training zone, slow down, and if you go under the lower end, work a bit harder.

At the gym, the cardiovascular (aerobic) equipment comes with built-in heart-rate monitors. For home you can buy portable monitors. Another way to gauge whether you're working within a suitable training zone is the 'perceived exertion test' – if you feel you're working but can still talk, then you're probably at a suitable intensity.

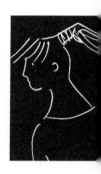

you and your health and fitness

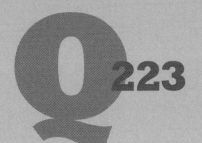

Q223

What's the best time to exercise to burn fat?

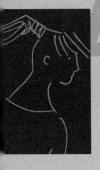

Studies on athletes show their peak time for training is in the evening, when body temperature, heart rate, reaction times and even flexibility are all 'at their best', so this is probably your best time to exercise as you may find it easier. One recent study found the hormones cortisol and thyrotropin were higher in exercisers at that time, indicating that the body is adapting better to training. Don't leave it too late – if you do anything other than winding-down yoga or stretching too close to bedtime, you may have trouble getting to sleep, as adrenalin levels may be high.

However, if you're an 'early bird', leaping out of bed full of energy, you could also use this time, after suitable warming up, to do some low-intensity aerobic work, like walking. Body fat may be burnt at a higher rate at this time (before you've had breakfast). Since you haven't eaten for 12 hours or so, the body can't use carbohydrates from a recent meal, so it tends to use fatty acids from the blood for energy.

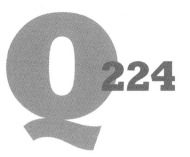

Q224

Which is best for weight control – weight training or aerobic exercise?

Most forms of aerobic exercise tend to burn more calories per minute than weight training and so, until recently, slimmers were advised to do a lot of aerobics and weight training was hardly mentioned. However, much recent research has concluded that weight training may be vital in slimming. Not only does it use calories while you are actually doing it, it raises metabolic rate afterwards, in a similar way to aerobic work.

Lastly, regular weight training increases lean tissue (muscle) and as muscle, even at rest, burns up more calories than body fat, it increases metabolic rate and helps you slim, or maintain weight. So the ideal exercise programme is one combining aerobic work and resistance training.

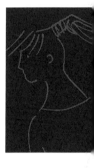

you and your health and fitness

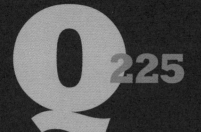

Q225

How does strength training help me lose weight?

A It can help to burn calories while you do it; it can raise your metabolic rate afterwards and can also raise your metabolic rate full-time, as your increased muscle mass, gained through the strength (weight/resistance) training, is more metabolically active than body fat.

I should also point out that if you add a lot of muscle through strength training you might actually find that you don't lose weight at all, even though you may alter your body composition and appear slimmer. The extra muscle weighs more than fat and so this effect may 'cancel out' the fat loss as far as weight goes. However, having a higher muscle percentage and lower body-fat percentage is great to aim for, as it makes you look slim and toned, and is healthier than being slim with a low lean tissue percentage – for example, you are at less risk of osteoporosis.

Q 226

Is it true that muscle converts into fat when you stop exercising?

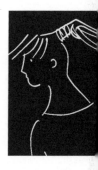

Muscle can't 'convert into' fat, as they're two completely different substances; muscle is mostly water and protein, whereas body fat is – well, fat. The body can convert surplus dietary fat, carbs or protein into fat if you eat too much. It can also do the reverse – use stored muscle and fat as energy, but it can't actually turn muscle into fat.

What may happen if you stop exercising is that muscles lose 'tone' and bulk. If, you continue eating as before, you'll create a calorie surplus, because without exercise and with decreased muscle, your body won't need so many calories to maintain its weight. Eventually surplus will be stored as fat – and there it is, muscle replaced with fat. However, definitely not, muscle 'converted' into fat by some bodily process, and the new fat won't necessarily appear in the same places as the muscle – it's more likely to end up around your waist.

To avoid this, the ex-exerciser needs to reduce calorie intake to meet new needs. Best of all – don't stop exercising, though sometimes it is inevitable, through injury, illness, etc.

Q227 Will isometrics get me slim?

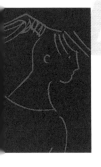

Isometrics are a static form of conditioning your muscles – normally a muscle is contracted and held for several seconds before being released. Done regularly, this can help you to look more toned up, as a floor-toning programme can, but it is it is not a major calorie-burning exercise, like aerobic activity or weight training. Yes, you'll burn a few extra calories doing it, but hardly enough to make any difference to your weight. Isometric exercise needs to be carried out properly and there is some evidence that it can increase blood pressure, so take advice from your gym or exercise teacher before using it to tone up.

Q228

Can you get fit and slim through gentle exercise, such as yoga?

Much yoga is deceptively not gentle and so, if you are looking for gentle exercise, be sure to check out your yoga class to make sure it really is that. Different kinds of yoga can be as relaxing or as tough as you want.

If you want gentle, you should join a beginners' hatha yoga class, for example. If you do it regularly, it will improve certain aspects of your fitness – particularly flexibility and perhaps strength. At any rate, you should find your body shape improving because yoga elongates the muscles and helps tone them. What gentle yoga won't do, though, is improve your cardiovascular fitness as it isn't aerobic, or build up a great deal of muscle, and therefore it won't burn many calories or increase your metabolic rate a great deal.

If you want to lose weight via exercise you need to couple aerobic work with strength training, as explained elsewhere.

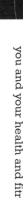

you and your health and fitness

301

Q229

How much weight can I expect to lose if I join the gym?

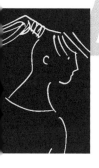

This depends on how often you go and what you do. Of the 16% of Britons who belong to a gym, less than half attend regularly! Let's say you go 2 to 3 times a week, however, and spend an average of 1 to 1½ hours using the equipment. Assuming 1 hour's cardiovascular work (e.g. treadmill, bike) and half an hour on resistance machines, you'd probably (depending on your weight, how hard you work, etc.) burn roughly 500 calories. So, you use 1,500 calories a week at the gym. As a pound of body fat equals about 3,500 calories, then you are, in theory, burning just under half a pound a week.

In my experience, though, new gym-goers very often lose less – nearer a pound a month. If unfit, it's hard to burn lots of calories per visit, at least in the first months. Of course, you'll be toning up and gradually building a little more muscle – so, over time, your body-fat percentage and figure should improve, as long as you go regularly and gradually increase times/distances/resistance, etc. The fitter you get, the more calories you'll burn.

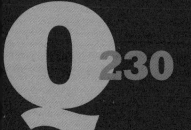

Q 230

Is there any exercise I should avoid if I'm very fat?

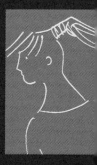

If you're very fat and also very unfit, then you should avoid all intense, hard, strenuous exercise and begin a gentle regime, such as 20 minutes' walking daily coupled with an easy body-toning programme of safe home exercise. Over time your fitness will improve and you can make the work you do harder.

In theory, fatness in itself – if you are healthy and fit – doesn't stop you doing any exercise, but in practice there are several activities that you would probably find uncomfortable – for example, jogging.

I would take your doctor's advice on what exercise to do other than that suggested above, and get a thorough health check-up at the same time. No doubt you should try to lose some weight, as diet and exercise do go together, and it makes little sense to get yourself fit if you are still carrying enough body fat to put your health at risk.

Q231

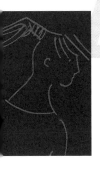

While exercising before a meal can help burn fat (Question 223), if prone to low-blood sugar or health problems this may not be wise as blood sugar levels can be low some time after your last meal and you could feel weak or faint. For normal exercise sessions (e.g. an hour's gym or average brisk walk), I'd suggest a healthy meal about 2 hours before, or a carb snack (with both quick- and slow-release carbs), about an hour before (say an apple and a banana). Anything too near exercise may cause you discomfort and affect performance.

During anything other than the mildest, shortest of activities, have a ready supply of water to keep hydrated (roughly 2 pints/1 litre per hour of moderate exercise) and drink plenty afterwards.

After long and/or strenuous exercise, you can have a snack of a quick-release carbohydrate (e.g. a banana or a slice of white bread and honey) to restore blood sugar. Slimmers note that after short or moderate exercise sessions, refuelling may not be necessary – you could end up taking in more calories than you've burnt.

you and your health and fitness

Q232

When is it unwise to exercise?

If you're ill you shouldn't exercise at all. If convalescing, get your doctor's advice. If you've done a lot of exercise in a short space of time, you should rest and give the body a chance to recuperate – overtraining damages the immune system and has other drawbacks.

Research at the University of Colorado found rats that exercised when they wanted to were healthier, with better immune systems, than rats forced to exercise against their wills. So, if you really aren't in the right frame of mind to exercise, perhaps it may be wise to leave it until later.

You should also exercise at a pace and intensity to match your current fitness – so attempting too hard an exercise is unwise. If you feel unusually tired after a workout, or have seriously aching muscles, then you've been over-exercising. It's also unwise to do high-intensity exercise infrequently – e.g. going to the gym after a month's absence and doing a hard workout on the Stairmaster. You may be risking a heart attack.

If you have long-term health problems, e.g. angina, or are pregnant, ask your doctor's advice before exercising.

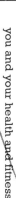

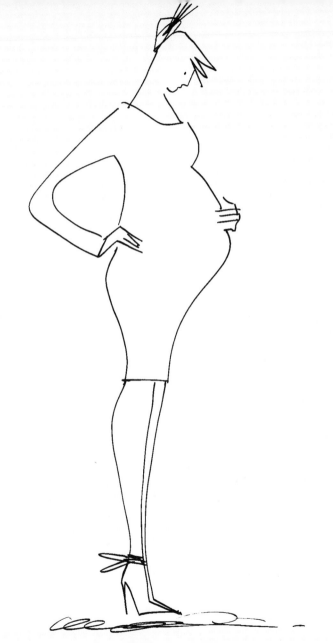

In the West, more women than men are obese, and it isn't hard to see why. It sometimes seems as though women have the odds stacked against them in their efforts to stay slim. They need to cope with the physiological fluctuations of monthly periods, most will experience pregnancy and lactation, and all will go through the menopause. All these affect the ability to stabilize weight.

While men don't have periods, pregnancy or the female menopause, nevertheless they do have plenty of stresses and problems of their own that can, and often do, influence their food and drink intake and therefore their weight and health.

Children are fatter than they have ever been. Look at the statistics – by age 15, according to the Obesity Resource Information Centre, 17.3% of girls and 16.4% of boys are obese, with many more overweight. 'The message is about saving lives.' In this chapter we look at ways of helping all the family to a slimmer, healthier future.

you and your special needs

Q233

However hard I try to lose weight, every month before my period I put on around 5 pounds. How can I avoid this?

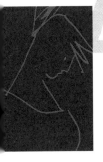

This is mostly fluid accumulating as a result of changes in levels of hormones. You'll notice you don't pass water as often in the days before your period. Some of the weight gain may also be due to constipation – again because the hormones tend to relax the colon muscles, so elimination isn't as efficient. You may also suffer from bloating through excess gas, once more because of hormones.

Once the period gets underway, the fluid is excreted, the constipation and bloating disappear, and everything should be back to normal – including your weight. Help with minimizing fluid retention appears in Question 238.

However, if you eat more than your body needs for fuel in the few days before your period as well, over time you may put on weight. If you think you're eating a lot more than normal at this time, see Questions 234–8. You do burn extra calories in the pre-menstrual period, so a little extra food won't put fat on you.

Women slimming shouldn't weigh themselves in the week before a period as this gain can make you depressed, even if you know it's not fat.

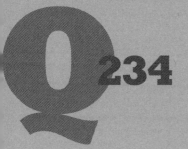

Q234

I tend to suffer from depression before my period is due, and this makes me comfort eat. What can I do about it?

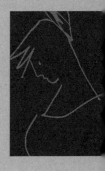

A healthy diet (all the time, not just in the days before your period) can help to alleviate PMS symptoms, including depression. Such a diet will include plenty of complex carbs, vitamin B-complex rich foods such as wholegrains, lean meat, fish, nuts, seeds, lentils and vegetables. Vitamin B6 is particularly linked with easing of PMS symptoms and is found in good amounts in fish, poultry, fortified breakfast cereals and nuts. There is also evidence that a diet rich in essential fatty acids (plant oils, oily fish), calcium (low-fat dairy produce, dark leafy greens, white fish) and magnesium (found in many of the foods listed already) can help minimize PMS symptoms, including depression.

The diet will also help regulate blood sugar levels and reduce the physical need to comfort eat. For more information on comfort eating and food cravings, see Questions 117, 140 and 235–8. It may also be an idea to see your doctor, who may be able to help in other ways – for example, going on the pill can minimize PMS and depression by altering hormone balance.

Q235

Before my period, I crave sweet foods, particularly chocolate. Why is this and what can I do about it?

As background, first read Questions 117 and 123, which give you general information on carbohydrate and chocolate cravings.

The reason that so many women do have cravings for sweet foods before a period is, it seems, usually because of the lack of circulating hormone oestrogen. Oestrogen is a 'stimulating' hormone for women, increasing production of serotonin (nature's Prozac), norepinephrine (noradrenaline) and endorphins (natural painkillers and pleasure-stimulators). Oestrogen is at its peak in your body at ovulation (mid-cycle) and at this time women often describe feeling particularly well and happy.

After ovulation, oestrogen levels decline quite rapidly and by the time the period is due they are at their lowest, and PMS is in full onslaught in many women. This may trigger the cravings for sweet foods – it could be the body's way of replacing the chemicals like serotonin, which will make you feel better. See also Question 237, which explains about the other female hormone, progesterone, and cravings.

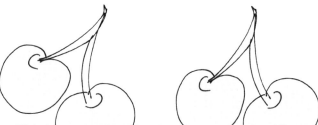

This is one explanation, but there could be others, and causes may vary from woman to woman. Production of insulin – the hormone regulating blood sugar levels – may also be affected by female hormonal fluctuations, adding to the 'chaos'.

One thing does seem to be certain – once you start giving in to the sweet food cravings, they are very difficult to control or stop. This is because the blood sugar levels may fluctuate (see Questions 67 and 68). Experts in PMS and diet advise eating 'little and often', using foods low on the Glycaemic Index (see Question 66) and high in fibre in the week or so before a period, as a good way to control sweet cravings at this time. Some examples of such snacks are: an apple and a dark rye crispbread; a pot of natural bio yoghurt and a few dried apricots; a pear and a few spoonfuls of baked beans. These snacks also have the benefit of offering a little natural sugar – fructose.

Some experts recommend chromium supplements, which some women find help ease the cravings, but there is no hard scientific evidence that these work, only anecdotal evidence. Never allow yourself to get too hungry at this time – and see Question 236 for an explanation of increased hunger pre-periods.

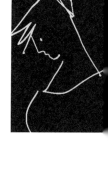

for women only

311

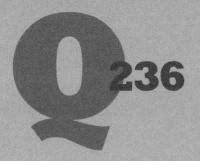

Q 236

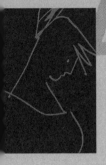

Questions 237 and 238 may help you understand cravings for carbs. However, many women, whether or not they get cravings, simply feel hungrier and eat bigger portions at meals before their periods, and then worry this will either cause weight gain or prevent weight loss if slimming.

There is a physiological reason for this – aided by the increase in progesterone, women's metabolic rates speed up after ovulation and before their period. This means you burn more calories and your body 'tells' you that you need more calories to cover this energy burst. You can tell your metabolic rate is increased because after ovulation you tend to feel hotter (wearing fewer layers or wanting the heat turned down). Average increased energy expenditure is thought to be around 250 calories a day, but it could be more.

So don't feel too bad when you find you're eating more before your period; unless you actually go completely overboard, it shouldn't hinder your diet or make you fat and therefore there is no need for a 'cure'. Follow the tips in the questions above on what and when to eat.

you and your special needs

312

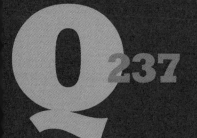

Q 237

At period time I crave carbs, particularly bread. Why is this?

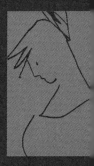

In pre-menstrual cravings, some women go for sweet foods (see Question 235), others high 'doses' of bread, potatoes and other starchy carbs – indeed, some crave both, but it's also likely fluctuating progesterone levels are at play.

After ovulation, progesterone increases until the body's sure it isn't pregnant, then levels drop rapidly until, just before the period's onset, levels of both it and oestrogen are low. (If pregnant, progesterone levels will remain high and, interestingly, it seems that, post-pregnancy, it's their sudden drop that may cause depression.)

Progesterone is the 'calming' hormone, as opposed to oestrogen's 'stimulating' properties, and just before your period your body may need an alternative source of 'calming'. Starches are the best foods for this effect.

Your doctor can advise you on therapy to help ease pre-menstrual hormonal upheaval. A good healthy diet can, however, go a long way towards easing the problem.

Avoid alcohol and coffee in the pre-menstrual phase, as these tend to worsen symptoms, and try to get your carbs from 'whole' sources, such as wholegrains, pulses, etc.

for women only

Q238 Before every period,
I swell up due to
fluid retention, which
makes me feel fat
and miserable. What
can I do about it?

Again, it's those female hormones at work here –
according to some experts, oestrogen tends to make the
body retain salt, which in turn means water retention. (At
any time of the month, if you eat a lot of salt your body
will retain extra water because it is literally trying to
dilute the extra salt to safe levels.) Other experts
believe that lack of vitamin B6 and/or magnesium, both
of which are important in retaining fluid balance, may
cause pre-menstrual fluid retention.

The truth is that we still don't know exactly what
causes PMS fluid retention in women (and why most
don't suffer from it). The fluid will probably become
most apparent in your breasts and abdomen and can
cause not only bloating and weight increase but also
pain, especially in the breasts (although not all pre-
menstrual breast pain is due to fluid retention).

You can help to minimize this fluid retention by eating
a low-salt diet and by avoiding foods containing highly
refined starches and sugars, such as cakes and biscuits,
which also contribute to fluid retention (the 'blotting

paper' syndrome). It is also wise to avoid all the salty, sugary, refined foods and drinks in any case, as they add little to your diet in terms of nutrition and, as we've seen in previous answers, such snacks can add to your premenstrual misery by making cravings and other symptoms worse. High insulin levels, stimulated by sugar, can cause more sodium retention, creating a vicious circle.

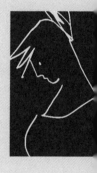

A diet rich in potassium will also help eliminate fluid – most fruits and vegetables contain good amounts of potassium. Foods rich in vitamin B6, magnesium, calcium, vitamin E and essential fatty acids may also help. You should also drink plenty of water, as this helps to dilute the salt – paradoxically, this won't increase the fluid retention. Although coffee is a diuretic, it's wise to avoid it at this time of the month as it can aggravate PMS symptoms, especially breast pain.

If you find it hard to cut right back on sugary and salty foods, try the retraining system outlined in Question 133. Don't take diuretic pills – long-term, they can actually increase the fluid retention problem and have other adverse effects.

Lastly, don't forget that a day or so after your period begins your body fluid level should return to normal. A healthy diet all month long will help the symptoms to be less severe next month.

Q239

Why do women naturally have much more body fat than men?

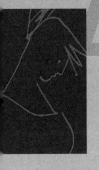

Women's extra fat has a purpose. A certain amount of fat is essential for ovulation and menstruation, and, therefore, in order to have children. If a woman's body-fat percentage drops below about 17% – and, indeed, if her BMI drops below about 18 – then she's at risk of losing her periods. Women tend to store fat on hips and thighs, which in past eras would supply long-term energy for pregnancy and breast-feeding when food supplies were uncertain.

Another reason why women have fat is to attract the male. Fat on the hips and thighs and breasts gives women the classic curvy 'hour-glass' figure that men are said to prefer. It is only in fairly recent times that thinness has been so sought after – and, even today, surveys show that a majority of men still prefer women not to be too slim. So, well-distributed fat has been nature's way of ensuring attraction and survival of the species.

Women's fat percentage and distribution seems to be governed by the hormone oestrogen – interestingly, when men take oestrogen as part of a sex-change process they develop extra fat on their hips and thighs.

Q240

Does sex burn off lots of calories?

If you let your partner do all the hard work, you probably won't burn more than an extra one or two calories a minute – little more than if sleeping. The actual orgasm only uses up a handful of calories.

If, however, you take a very active role, you may well burn an extra 6 or 7 calories a minute. Of course, the total amount will depend on how long sex lasts. As the average is a rather meagre 4 minutes, I think we can safely say that, active or not, sex isn't going to help lose much weight. One four-minute session, including orgasm, would burn only enough calories to cancel out one rye crispbread. A brisk walk is a much better idea, because it's bound to last longer.

However, regular (say, at least 3 times a week) sex may bring some other small benefits. During sex, your body manufactures chemicals similar to those released when you eat chocolate and carbohydrates. Therefore, if you're the kind of person who tends to binge, regular sex may reduce this need. Sex and orgasms also help flatten the stomach, by working abdominal muscles.

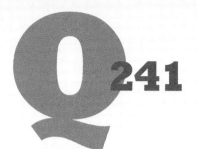

Q241

What is cellulite and is it caused by toxins?

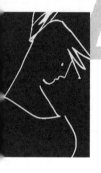

Cellulite is the, sometimes dimpled, appearance of fat on women's bottoms, hips or thighs. Cellulite fat is similar scientifically to 'normal' fat. The dimpled appearance is, however, not a figment of women's imaginations and, although still debated, the explanation seems to be that women's fat cells are grouped in sacs held between the skin's tissue layers by vertical fibrous strands of connective tissue. These cannot expand, so – especially when weight is gained or the skin squeezed – the fat globules push through, producing the orange-peel look.

Oestrogen causes women to lay down most fat on their bottoms, hips and thighs – where 'cellulite' is most obvious. Poor skin tone/elasticity, and lack of exercise don't help.

Although many 'therapists' will provide 'detoxing' diet cures, there's no scientific evidence that cellulite is caused by toxins. If detox regimes help it look better, it's usually because they're low in calories and result in weight loss, including some fat and fluid from the offending areas. The subject is also usually required to follow other strategies, including exercise and massage, which may help.

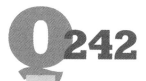

Q242 Why don't men get cellulite?

Men's connective tissue is, apparently, formed differently from women's (see Question 241 opposite), with the result that fat cells don't bulge through in the same way. Also, male hormones dictate that, in men, fat usually tends to be laid down in the abdominal area and trunk rather than on the hips and thighs. Lastly, men's outer skin is much thicker and provides a firmer layer so that subcutaneous fat is less noticeable.

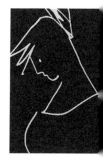

Q243 Why do even slim women get cellulite?

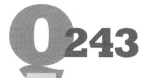

Even a slim woman has a body-fat composition of around 20% fat and, as we have discussed, women's natural oestrogen means that fat is often deposited on the bottom, hips and thighs, where the cellulite (see Question 241) appears. Skin tone, strength and elasticity may also be poor, and this may increase with age, hence older slim women are more likely to suffer from cellulite than young ones. However, slim women who take a lot of regular lower-body exercise (e.g. runners, dancers, ice-skaters) very rarely have any signs of cellulite.

for women only

Q244

How can I get rid of cellulite?

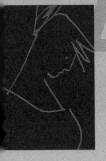

Diet, exercise and massage. A reduced-calorie diet will help create a calorie deficit and shift the fat forming the cellulite. However, no diet can make fat disappear from your lower body only – you'll lose fat from elsewhere too. Exercise will also help burn calories and shift the fat; and lower body exercise, like cycling, walking, and toning exercises, will improve the appearance of the cellulite. Lastly, field trials show regular vigorous massaging of the skin above the cellulite (using, for example, a loofah and an inexpensive moisturizing cream) may also improve its appearance.

This combined effort will show results if kept up long enough, but don't expect fast results. When the body loses fat, it goes first from the abdomen and upper body, and last from the lower body. In this respect, women are again at a disadvantage, as the female body may try harder to 'hang on' to its lower-body fat. Think in terms of six months and plenty of effort and you won't be disappointed.

Q245

I'd like to become pregnant soon, but I'm very overweight. Does this matter?

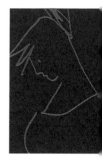

To some extent it depends on exactly how overweight you are. If very obese, you may be advised to slim down to a BMI under 30. Overweight women are more likely to suffer from diabetes or high blood pressure during pregnancy and there may also be other problems, like increased risk of back pain, varicose veins and haemorrhoids.

It is also in your interest not to be obese if you want to conceive soon, as there is evidence, according to the British Nutrition Foundation, that 'excessive stores of body fat can impair fertility', and women with a BMI over 30 have a lower pregnancy rate than those with a BMI under 20.

Go back to Question 26 and work out your BMI. If it is over 30, see your doctor and discuss your weight with him or her.

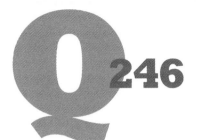

Q246 Should I eat for two when pregnant?

The UK Dietary Reference values for pregnancy suggest that, on average, women need only an extra 200 cals/day during the last 3 months of pregnancy. Other expert guidelines suggest up to an extra 300 cals/day during the last 4–5 months. Almost every woman is different and these can be but guidelines. The best approach is to 'follow your appetite' (using common sense – I use the word 'appetite' in its real meaning) and if you're gaining weight roughly according to advice you've received (read Question 249), you're doing fine.

This means you don't need to 'eat for two' – if you mean doubling calorie intake! Certainly, in the first few months of pregnancy you hardly need eat any extra at all. This is even more pertinent if you start overweight – these early months are an ideal time to ensure you don't put on more, over the whole pregnancy, than absolutely necessary for a healthy baby.

Research shows that in pregnancy the body adapts to conserve energy, especially if you don't eat enough, by slowing down thyroid gland activity. And at this time the foetus is so small it doesn't need many calories – rather, it needs nutrients for growth and health. Also, towards the end of pregnancy the mother is naturally less active and calories are conserved that way, too. Lastly, when you're pregnant the gastrointestinal system becomes more efficient at absorbing nutrients.

When you do begin to eat more in the last half of the pregnancy, as a guide, 250–300 extra calories a day can be covered by one of the following:

• An average chicken salad sandwich.
• Increasing portion sizes of breakfast, lunch and main meal by 15% (one sixth).
• A large (90g/3^{1}/4oz) slice of fruit cake.
• A medium (225g/8oz) baked potato with baked bean topping.
• 250ml (9fl oz) semi-skimmed milk and 1 large slice of bread with low-fat spread and Marmite. As you can see, the extra doesn't amount to a great deal.

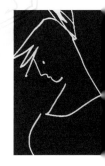

There is also evidence to indicate that the last thing you should do is to increase intake of saturated fats – found in greatest quantities in full-fat dairy produce, fatty meat and many processed sweet and savoury snacks. Research at St Thomas's Hospital, London, in 2000 found that a diet high in saturated fat increased the blood cholesterol levels in the foetus, creating an increased risk of the baby later developing heart disease and diabetes.

So what is most important during your pregnancy is that you get a healthy, varied, balanced diet rich in all the nutrients needed by your growing baby, as advised by your pre-natal dietitian.

for women only

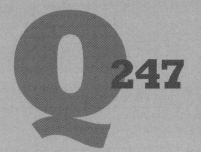

Q247

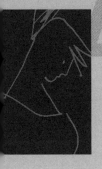

Why do you want to lose weight during pregnancy? If seriously overweight, you could lose weight before conceiving – the most sensible way of tackling a weight problem, for both you and the baby.

If you find yourself pregnant and seriously overweight, you should see your doctor or pre-natal clinic dietitian for advice. Although there are several possible health problems associated with 'maternal obesity' during pregnancy, it's uncommon for women to be prescribed a strict reduced-calorie diet during pregnancy. A 13lb (6kg) gain is the minimum recommended for obese women.

If slightly overweight when you first become pregnant – say, with a BMI of around 26–9, you'll probably be advised simply to monitor your weight and try to put on no more than the recommended lower amount of gain – 15–25lb (7–11.5kg) – during pregnancy. If not overweight, welcome pregnancy weight gain as a sign baby is healthy.

Don't follow any kind of calorie-restricted diet during pregnancy without advice from those who have your case notes and can monitor you in person.

you and your special needs

324

Q248

The average total weight it's wise to gain is described in the next question. If you were an average weight (BMI 20–25) at the start of pregnancy, after the first 3 months you should gain, on average, no more than about 1lb (0.5kg) a week until the last 4 weeks, when weight often stabilizes. If you are gaining much more, it's wise to go for a check-up straight away. The weight gain may be fluid, which requires medical advice.

If you know you're eating a lot more than usual (and definitely more than the extra 300 cals/day outlined), this could be the reason for weight gain. Cut down on fatty, sugary foods and substitute complex carbs, like wholemeal bread and potatoes, fruit and, to a lesser extent, nuts, seeds and lean fish or chicken. If ravenous between meals, snack on fruit, rye crispbreads, or similar.

Talk to your specialist about your fears – they should weigh you regularly anyway and advise you even without your asking. Above average weight gain shouldn't negatively affect baby's health.

for women only

Q249

What is the right amount of weight to gain during pregnancy?

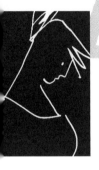

You need to gain enough to ensure optimum weight, health and nutrition for the baby, but not so much you have an uncomfortable pregnancy and/or complications, and aren't left with much fat to lose afterwards.

Recommendations for weight gain are usually based on those from the USA National Academy of Sciences Food and Nutrition Board: 24–36lb (11.5–1kg) for conception BMIs of 20–25.9, 15–25lb (7–11.5kg) for BMIs of 26–29, and 13lb (6kg) for BMIs of 30 and over (ideals for optimum baby health and least risk to it).

Foetus, placenta and other essentials weigh about 20–22lb (9–10kg); the remaining gain is fat. Research shows that although high weight gain in pregnancy may be associated with more complications, prolonged labour and retained maternal weight, it appears not to affect the baby adversely – rather, the baby may have an above-average birth-weight, which may not be a disadvantage.

On average, most gain occurs in months 4 to 8. A gain of 3lb (1.35kg) or so is adequate in the first 3 months; after that about 1lb (0.5kg) a week until week 36 is about right.

you and your special needs

326

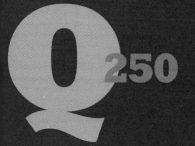

Q250

If an average baby weighs about 8lb, can't I just put on 8lb so when the baby is born I will be my correct weight?

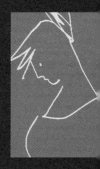

AWeight gained isn't just the baby. About 20–22lb (9–10kg) 'essential' weight is in items over and above fat you may put on. After birth, you lose about 10–13lb (4.5–6kg) from baby, amniotic fluid and placenta. In the next few days more pounds go as extra fluids and blood normalize. The uterus (womb) gradually shrinks too; so in about another 2 weeks you should have lost most extra 'essential' weight.

Most women also put on some fat. Although, as research shows laying down fat in pregnancy isn't essential for baby (it takes what it needs from mother), maternal fat deposition is encouraged by increase in progesterone, the body's way of ensuring food for baby after its birth (mother will make breast milk from her fat stores). At an average gain of 30lb (13.75kg), maternal fat deposits would be about 10lb (4.5kg); enough to breast-feed baby for the first 10 weeks!

By eating very carefully during pregnancy you could limit extra gain to less than 10lb, but don't consider low-calorie dieting. Breast-feeding is a much better way to get your figure back.

Q251

If I crave particular foods when pregnant does my body need their nutrients?

Most pregnant women 'go off' certain foods and develop a strong taste for others – normally called having 'cravings' – which may be for basic ordinary foods such as oranges, or for more unusual items like caviar or dill pickles! Cravings for non-food items, such as coal, are called pica.

If you crave fatty, salty or sugary foods during pregnancy, it is best to try to control these cravings, using techniques described in Questions 117–127 and 234–7 for non-pregnant women. These types of foods don't supply good quantities of the essential nutrients you and the baby need, and also tend to be high in calories and perhaps saturated fat (see Question 246).

It isn't true that all cravings are a result of your body needing the nutrients they contain – as we've seen, a lot of craved foods contain hardly any nutrients at all except calories. Although some believe that cravings are linked to nutritional need, there is little scientific evidence that any craving is based on a physical requirement for a particular nutrient. If you crave 'pica' non-foods, talk to your doctor.

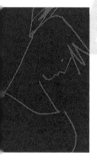

you and your special needs

Q 252

Is plenty of exercise the best way to keep weight down during pregnancy or should I just put my feet up and avoid exercise?

You don't really want to keep your weight down, you want to gain approximately the recommended amount. If you see exercise as a way to ensure you don't put on too much weight, though, you're partly right. Regular suitable exercise can help keep you fit and a reasonable weight. It does depend, though, on your definition of 'plenty'.

More vigorous types of exercise – like jogging or gym work – become increasingly difficult in the later stages of pregnancy, and may actually be detrimental to foetal bone composition. It's better to cut exercise down to small easy sessions rather than long calorie-burning bouts.

If you've only done mild or moderate exercise before, though, you shouldn't suddenly do a lot more when pregnant. Walking and swimming are probably the ideal forms of calorie-burning exercise for pregnancy.

Take advice from your pre-natal clinic on the best forms of exercise for you – essential if you have a history of miscarriage and/or any problems in early pregnancy.

Some women do use pregnancy as an excuse to do little and eat plenty, but live to regret it after the birth.

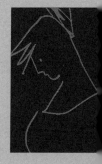

for women only

Q253

When my baby is born what's the best way to get my figure back and how soon can I begin exercising?

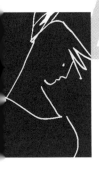

Breast-feeding is ideal for creating a small calorie deficit so you gradually lose surplus pounds (see Question 256). Breast-feeding also contracts the uterus to normal quickly, has many health benefits for the baby and is convenient, so it's strongly recommended. Whether breast-feeding or not, you don't need high-fat, high-sugar and/or high-salt snacks, so cut right back on them.

If you had a non-Caesarean delivery, you should walk around a little within hours, to improve circulation. In the first day or two, you can do very gentle exercise to get your stomach muscles working again (see Question 254) and gradually increase the walking.

Once home, carry on walking, say taking the baby briefly out twice daily. You can begin an exercise programme a week after the birth, taking it gently and stopping if anything hurts. Also remember posture, as this'll quickly help you get your figure back.

If you've had a bikini-incision Caesarean, delay all this until after 3 weeks; if an 'up and down', wait until the 6-week check-up before beginning a full exercise programme.

you and your special needs

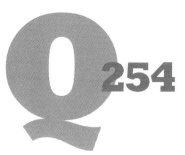

Q254

What is the best exercise to get my stomach back into shape after the birth?

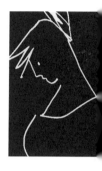

Unless you've had a Caesarean, do these in the first week:

1 First day, lie on back with pillow under head and knees bent, feet flat on bed/floor. Slowly extend legs until straight out. Draw one back in slowly, trying to feel stomach muscles working, then draw in other. Repeat once or twice, twice a day, gradually building to 10.
2 Lie as before but with legs out straight but relaxed, arms at sides. Lift left leg up and over right to touch left heel on bed/floor next to right leg. Try to feel stomach muscles working. Slowly move leg back and repeat with right. Repeat once or twice, gradually building up to 10.

Later, if up to it, do curl-ups. Make them as easy as you like – as long as done regularly, your muscles will gradually strengthen and you can come up further.

After six-week check-up, if you still have a 'tummy', some of it may be fat, see Questions 255–6. You can also add in some hill walking and swimming. Remember, breast-feeding is great for shrinking your stomach back.

for women only

Q255

I need to lose weight but I'm breast-feeding. How can I slim safely?

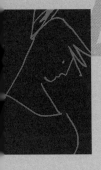

As breast-feeding uses around 500 cals/day for the first 4 months of sole feeding, you'll lose weight gradually if you eat the same number of cals/day as you would to maintain weight if not breast-feeding. For most this is around 2,000. On such a gentle, safe diet, breast milk won't dry up.

The main thing to ensure is that when you are, in effect, reducing your breast-feeding diet by 500 calories a day, it's not at the expense of nutrients your baby needs. One good way to ensure this is to cut out high-fat, high-sugar and/or high-salt items, such as biscuits, sweets, crisps, etc. Get a healthy diet with plenty of fruit and veg, complex carbs, lean protein (red meat is good), fish, and plenty of essential fats, so vital for the baby's brain development. Also drink plenty of water.

See how you get on with this for 2 weeks – if you're losing weight gradually, the baby is thriving, and you don't feel hungry, you can probably continue down to a suitable weight. Talk your diet through with your doctor or post-natal dietitian if you have worries.

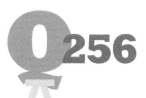

Q256

If not breast-feeding, what calorie intake do I aim for to slim?

Use Question 85 to work out how many calories a day you need to lose weight and follow whichever plan suits you, using Questions 82–5 and 93–4. When busy with a new baby, you need a simple diet, so low-fat might be best, or the traffic light plan (Question 95). Don't try to lose weight too quickly; you need good nutrition when stressed (new mothers are).

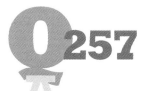

Q257

Does HRT cause weight gain?

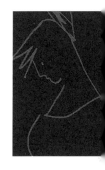

As you'll see in the next question, recent studies found no link between weight gain and HRT. One large study actually found women on HRT during and after the menopause maintained a slightly lower weight than those not. In some women, HRT does cause fluid retention, which can make the body look larger, but this isn't fat.

A low-salt diet, high in fruits and veg, can help minimize fluid retention. If putting on weight with HRT – fluid or fat – a different formulation may help. You may also find natural progesterone cream (prescription only in the UK) helps hot flushes, etc. without causing fluid retention.

for women only

Q258 Is weight gain inevitable for a woman during and after menopause?

Despite the fact so many women say they gain weight during the menopausal years, recent studies – particularly two important US ones – have concluded that neither the perimenopause (the years immediately before menses cease), menopause nor HRT is the cause of weight gain.

The conclusions from studying hundreds of women from 17 years before to 22 years after menopause, were that from about 35–65, women gain total body weight gradually and steadily, and neither loss of ovarian hormones nor their HRT replacement makes a detectable difference.

The World Health Organization agrees – its obesity report in 2001 said most weight gain associated with menopause has been attributed to reduced activity. The US studies concluded that although many women gain weight during menopause this is part of a 'bigger picture' of gain of around 0.43% per year during midlife. For a 10 stone (64kg) woman this represents under 1lb (0.5kg) a year.

In fact, in one of the trials, about 3 years after onset of menopause there was an average 3% weight loss in the women studied – a blip researchers couldn't explain. It does, therefore, seem that you don't have to gain weight over the menopause, but that most women do slowly gain weight throughout middle age, due to the slowing down of the metabolic rate and a typical lack of physical activity.

So, if weight gain in midlife is probably not associated with menopause, is it still inevitable during the 'mid' decades? Even in fit people, a small change in body shape does seem to happen (see Question 23), but large gains can be kept at bay with a sensible diet, resistance exercise to blunt muscle loss and aerobic exercise to burn calories.

As one of the US studies says, a powerful predictor of elevated BMI (increased weight) was physical inactivity – suggesting the most useful intervention for preventing weight gain in midlife women is increasing activity.

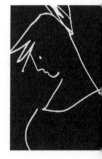

So why do so many women say they've piled on weight over the menopause? Experts say lowered oestrogen levels tend to redistribute body fat, increasing deposits around the waist, while legs and arms may get thinner. Therefore dress size will increase, and women taking synthetic progesterone as part of HRT may suffer from fluid retention. Others become very tired or have other adverse symptoms, which make it harder for them to feel motivated to exercise. Comfort eating may also be a factor.

Although there seems to be no evidence to prove it, I don't doubt that some women do gain weight over the menopausal period, over and above the 'normal' slow midlife increase. After all, the figures quoted in the research are based on averages not individuals. Plumper women tend to produce more oestrogen after menopause and some experts believe this may encourage weight gain.

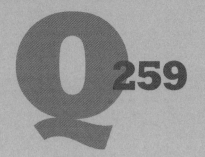

Is it true that
midlife weight gain
for a woman is
healthy?

This is partially true. If you try to maintain too low a
body weight during midlife you may predispose
yourself to reduced bone mass and higher risk of
osteoporosis. This is partly because body fat helps
retain stores of oestrogen, loss of which is a major factor
in post-menopausal bone loss. Low body weight also
generally means lower bone density – thin people have
less bone mass on average than heavier ones. It's also
been said that plump women tend to have fewer
menopausal problems, though I can't find research to
back this up.

Those are two good reasons not to aim to maintain too
low a body weight in midlife. A BMI in the upper range
of 'healthy' (i.e. nearer 25) may be prudent. A good rule-
of-thumb is that if you were very slim in your youth and
20s, you shouldn't worry if you put on a stone or so by
around 50 – it is probably doing you more good than
harm, especially if you exercise regularly.

However, it isn't healthy to gain too much weight.
Elsewhere you can see the long list of health risks

you and your special needs

associated with overweight. A recent study found 'middle-aged' women were much more likely to suffer from 'Syndrome X'. This is a 'clustering' factor of five overweight-related symptoms, including insulin resistance and the pre-diabetic state, two or more of which can act in combination to increase the risk of cardiovascular disease significantly. The conclusion was that women should avoid midlife weight gain. Obesity in post-menopausal women is also linked with increased risk of breast cancer, high blood pressure, heart disease and arthritis of the weight-bearing joints.

The message seems to be that weight gain in midlife should be kept small, BMI should be kept within reasonable bounds (if yours is over 28 you may have cause for concern) and a programme of healthy eating and exercise should be undertaken to facilitate all this.

for women only

Q260

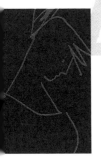

Yes, many women have successfully lost or stabilized weight during this time. In recent research scientists have not found any actual physiological reason why weight gain (or difficulty in losing it) should be associated with menopause, (see Questions 258 and 259). The best strategy is to increase regular exercise output, while choosing a healthy slimming diet.

As you age, metabolic rate generally decreases slowly and you need to work a bit harder to keep it 'stoked up' through exercise. A combination of resistance and aerobic exercise works best. As weight tends to increase around the abdomen and waist during menopause, and arms and legs get thinner, it'll also improve overall shape.

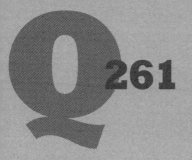

Q 261

My body seems to have slowed down since menopause. Is this possible and what can I do about it?

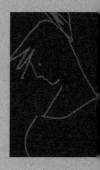

There is a natural and fairly inevitable 'slowing down' as one ages. Although this can be blunted with determination, regular exercise to improve strength, suppleness and aerobic capacity, and a happy and inquisitive outlook, it's asking a bit too much that you keep everything in 100% condition. This may partly account for your feeling that you're slowing down. In your 50s or 60s, however, you shouldn't feel 'old'. A fit 60-year-old can be as fit as the average 35-year-old.

Some menopausal symptoms, like generalized aches and pains, and tiredness – can make you feel less likely to stride out as you used to. If this is the case, things should get back to normal afterwards, although it can take time.

Make an effort to hurry when you find yourself dawdling; write a plan for a regular exercise schedule to improve circulation; breathe deeply to oxygenate body and brain. Find interesting things to do – people walk slowly when not interested in the destination, but hurry when there's something of interest. Get a check-up in case of medical problems and eat a healthy diet.

for women only

Q 262

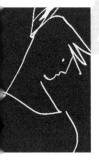

Over 35, our metabolic rate gradually slows, and this is progressive, so at, say, 70 you will burn about 350 cals/day less than you did at 35 (the equation is an average of 50 cals/day less for every 5 years of your life). So, if you don't want to put on weight, you either have to eat a little less or exercise more. The advice for people in their 50s and 60s is roughly the advice to anyone – cut down on 'junk'-type foods like high-fat, high-sugar, high-salt processed snacks, etc. eat as healthy and varied a diet as you can, and (with your doctor's permission) increase exercise as much as you're able, depending on health and circumstances. Maintaining a reasonable weight in mid and later life is one of the best ways to stay healthy.

As you get older – into the 70s or 80s – many find the appetite diminishes and the digestive system becomes slightly more difficult to please, which will alter your eating patterns. If you have any nutrition, eating or digestive worries, or want to begin exercising, see your doctor.

you and your special needs

340

Q 263

Is it ever too late to start a diet? My mother is 75 and very overweight.

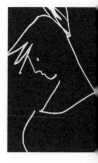

There's no reason why someone of 75 (or older) shouldn't reduce calorie intake and lose weight, but it's best done with the help of a doctor or dietitian who knows them. It's often hard to persuade older people to diet – many resist change and their system may not welcome new foods. So dietary changes need monitoring, even if acceptable to them. The advice to 'take exercise' often can't apply to obese elderly people because they can't. If weight is lost, mobility should increase.

If your mother is obese, she should be being monitored by her doctor, who should make the decisions about her diet. Even losing 5% weight can make a big difference to risk of related health problems. So it would be good if she can lose some – but she has to be happy with changes.

Nutritional requirements for old people are the same, apart from reduction in calories and a requirement for vitamin D (cod liver oil is the easiest source) if she doesn't get outdoors much. Even if you only ensure she cuts down high-fat, high-sugar snacks, it may help her weight and nutritional status.

for women only

Q 264

Is there any difference between the type of diet a man should follow for weight loss and that for a woman?

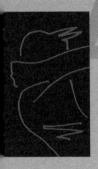

On average, men have higher metabolic rates than women – because they're heavier, with a higher percentage of lean tissue. Therefore men need more calories on their reduced-calorie diets; otherwise they'll feel too hungry and lose weight too quickly. Questions 2–5 will help you calculate your metabolic rate and Question 85 help you decide what calorie intake you should aim for.

Apart from that, men and women can follow the same types of diet. People with a higher metabolic rate will simply increase portion sizes, giving them more nutrients across the board. Some men may need a little more protein – for example, men who do hard physical work or professional sportsmen. Indeed, the male affinity with protein may explain why research shows they tend to lose weight best on a high-protein diet like a modified Atkins.

However, men reading this probably won't be sportsmen or highly active. Most men who need to diet have been taking too little physical activity long-term, and even starting a moderate activity programme are unlikely to need much extra protein, at least in the early months.

Q265

I'm overweight, but as alcohol helps prevent heart disease in men, shouldn't I carry on drinking and cut down calories elsewhere?

Drinking just one glass of red wine or dark beer a day is enough to help prevent heart disease and provide other health protection, so you can cut all the rest of your drinking out as an obvious and easy way to save calories without having to worry that your health will suffer.

More than four units a day is likely to cause you more health problems than benefits. Although alcohol has a few trace nutrients in it, by and large it is 'empty calories' and you would be much, much better off cutting back on that than on healthy nutritious foods if you want to save calories. In fact, if you don't want to drink alcohol at all, a glass of red grape juice will have a similar protective effect to the red wine; it contains the beneficial polyphenols found in the grapes.

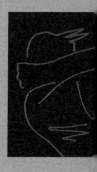

You will find more information about alcohol and overweight in Questions 168, 169 and 267, and more information on a healthy diet in Chapter Two.

for men only

343

Q266 I'm not overweight but I've put 4 inches on my waist in the last 10 years. I am 50. Is this normal – and reversible?

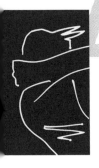

This is the typical male pattern of weight gain – the 'apple' effect, discussed elsewhere. For men, any small gain in adulthood tends to gather around the abdomen and waist, at any age. The thickening waist for men is also compounded by poor posture (the middle may literally 'sag', as the area between hips and ribcage is supported only by muscle) and by lack of specific exercise for the midriff. Studies show that even very fit men increase girth by around 2 inches (5cm) as they get older, so there is some inevitability about it – but it can be minimized if you are determined enough.

For most men, however, 4 inches (10cm) is quite a lot to gain in 10 years and I would guess you have put on some weight. I expect you've also given up most forms of exercise that may keep your midriff toned. Set aside regular time to exercise all your stomach muscles, and consider losing a few pounds, which will almost certainly go from your stomach and waist first, through watching what you eat and taking more aerobic exercise.

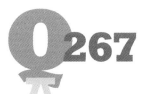

Q267

Does beer drinking really cause a 'beer belly'?

As seen in Question 62, consuming a diet high in simple carbs can tend to put fat on people around the midriff rather than other areas. Beer (along with wine, lager, cider, etc.) can be classed as a simple carb and thus its not inconsiderable calories may indeed arrive on your belly first. But that isn't the whole picture – a pint (200 calories for standard beer) can be factored into anyone's daily ration, but if you regularly have several pints you'll probably be getting many more calories than you need and thus, just as if you ate a couple too many chocolate bars, you can put on weight through drinking.

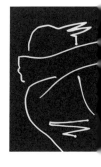

Q268

When I gain weight, why does it always go to my belly first?

Men tend to be 'apple-shaped', women 'pear-shaped', thanks to the differing patterns of fat laying-down due to different hormone levels. So, in most men weight naturally gravitates towards the stomach. There's also evidence that stress can increase abdominal fat (see Question 195), so try to de-stress. The good news is that the 'belly' seems to contain a type of fat easier to disperse than fat elsewhere.

for men only

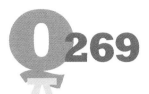

Q269

Is a pot belly a cause for concern?

A large 'pot' is worrying because it is more closely linked with health problems than is fat elsewhere. Indeed, some experts believe that waist circumference (and 'pot') is more important than your actual weight in predicting future health risks. Other parts of the book explain this in more detail.

Q270

How do I slim my pot belly but keep the rest of my shape?

If you're a little overweight and follow a calorie-reduced diet for a few weeks you should find that the fat goes from your stomach more noticeably than from other places, as the typical 'pot belly' seems to contain a type of fat much easier to disperse than fat elsewhere. You should also do exercises for the midriff to tone you up and make the stomach look slimmer.

you and your special needs

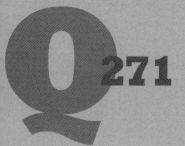

Q271

Can I do anything about my embarrassing flabby 'breasts'? I'm not very fat, but I get teased about them.

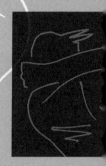

The name for this is gynaecomastia – meaning the over-development of breast tissue in males. Being overweight is normally the cause – you don't have to be obese to notice the syndrome, but I would guess that you're probably at least 1 or 2 stone(s) overweight, with a typical male 'apple shape'. (Check out your BMI as explained in Question 26.)

What happens is the fatty tissue produces the female hormone oestrogen, which stimulates development of fat in the breast area. If you lose weight all over you'll reduce oestrogen levels and the 'breasts' will reduce in size.

You should also cut right back on alcohol if you've been a heavy drinker. Alcohol abuse reduces the ability of the liver to break down complex steroid hormones and can make gynaecomastia worse. Low levels of testosterone in the body may also contribute to breast development – you should see your doctor and, if a test shows this is the case, he may offer supplements.

Lastly, regular exercises to strengthen the pectoral muscles should also help.

for men only

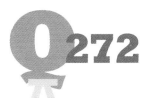

Q272

Are there fat-burning exercise classes not aimed at women?

A recent survey of exercise classes found that you are most likely to meet fellow males at boxercise classes or Ashtanga yoga classes. Boxercise is no surprise, although apparently 40% of devotees are female. You may be amazed to learn that you can burn fat through yoga, but Ashtanga is fast and furious and quite hard.

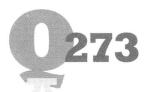

Q273

I dislike the gym and outdoor exercise. How do I burn calories?

There are various things you can do at home – for example, skipping (an excellent, quick way to burn calories and get fit), or using a mini-trampoline, exercise bike, treadmill or rowing machine. You could also pursue indoor sports such as badminton, tennis, squash, or swimming. I suppose you're including walking in your list of outdoor activities you dislike, but if you hadn't thought of walking as an outdoor exercise, it really is an excellent calorie-burning activity, especially if you're not very fit to begin with. To make it more purposeful, you could do what many have done before and get a dog.

Q274 Is there a male menopause and if so is it the cause of my weight gain?

It seems there is a male menopause, which could have various side effects, including weight gain. According to studies in 2001, there's an average decrease in levels of the male hormone testosterone in midlife males, starting at a similar age to female menopause – around 50. This can cause not only weight gain, loss of muscle mass and energy, but also depression, mood swings, lowered sex drive, memory loss and irritability. Low testosterone levels seem to reduce blood supply to the brain, meaning a general slowing of the metabolism.

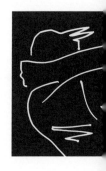

As with women, symptoms vary from man to man and may be slight or severe. If you feel this may be your problem, see your doctor. Development is underway in male HRT, which may also include the female hormone oestrogen, found to protect men against osteoporosis and also possibly against mental decline and memory loss.

Meanwhile, sensible eating and increasing aerobic and resistance exercise will help minimize symptoms. The bonus is that with healthy diet and more exercise you're also giving yourself natural protection against old age.

for men only

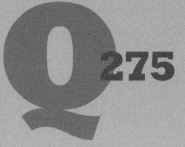

Q 275 How do I tell if my child is overweight and how important IS overweight in children?

A Believe it or not, there is no national or international consensus on the precise definition of overweight and obesity in children. For several years, doctors have been inclined to use 'percentile' weight for age charts, which need to be interpreted on an individual basis, taking into account the child's height – obviously if your child is much heavier than average but also much taller than average, then he or she may not be overweight at all.

However, in 2000 a British team from the Institute of Child Health with the International Obesity Task Force produced a set of international cut-off points for overweight and obesity in children based on the Body Mass Index (see Question 26). This produces guidelines for children based on their weight and height from age 2 to 18, after which the standard BMI charts are used. These cut-off points correspond to an adult BMI of 25+ for overweight and, although they have not yet been taken on board internationally, many experts believe that they offer the best assessment of overweight in children.

According to these, your child is overweight if he/she is:

Age	with a BMI more than		Age	with a BMI more than	
2	18.4	18	11	20.6	20.7
3	17.9	17.6	12	21.2	21.7
4	17.6	17.3	13	21.9	22.6
5	17.4	17.1	14	22.6	23.3
6	17.6	17.3	15	23.3	23.9
7	17.9	17.8	16	23.9	24.4
8	18.4	18.3	17	24.5	24.7
9	19.1	19.1	18	25	25
10	19.8	19.9			
	Boys	Girls		Boys	Girls

Some experts also suggest simply looking at your child with the rest of his/her class at school and seeing if he/she seems much bigger than most of the others as a reasonable way to tell if there is a weight problem. It is also advisable to see your doctor, who will no doubt be able to add a professional opinion and further advice.

As to how important overweight is in children, we're facing an obesity epidemic that looks set to get worse unless we act quickly. The main problem is that studies show that a high percentage of children/adolescents become fat adults, with the health implications that brings.

There are not many truly fat children who go on to be slim adults, so it's obviously much better to prevent overweight in your child as a way to combat adult obesity. And, if your child has become overweight, the sooner you do something about it, the easier it should be to resolve.

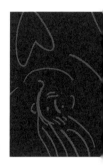

for kids (and parents) only

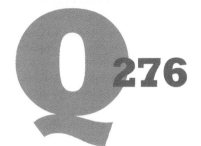

Q276 What's the best way to prevent a child from becoming overweight?

Getting your kids to eat well is perceived as a sign of being a 'good parent'. For many children, though, a healthy appetite for decent food is but a short trip to a big appetite for all kinds of food, followed by the first signs of overweight. Encourage your child to eat well – but that doesn't mean overeating.

It's also important to eat sensibly yourself. Research shows overweight tends to run in families, as does amount of exercise taken. Overweight may be partially due to genetic predisposition (Question 12) but, even so, children tend to take eating habits from parents and older siblings, and if what's offered is healthy and balanced, reasonably low in fat and sugar, then the child is unlikely to get fat, especially if encouraged to do lots of physical activity. Take your child hiking, swimming, cycling – help him/her to join sports clubs.

Sadly, school PE and sports are tending to be sidelined by curriculum demands, so may not offer as much exercise as it did. A 2005 US report on activity levels of over 2000 children aged 10 to 18, found exercise declined drastically during this period and corresponded exactly with increases in their BMI. So it's important to develop your child's awareness of physical activity by encouraging her/him at every opportunity. Lead by example – and keep slim and fit yourself!

You need to take an active interest in what your child eats. Research shows modern children tend to eat a great deal of 'snack' foods both outside and in the home. Many have access to a 'snacks' cupboard and a fridge stocked full with crisps, fizzy drinks and so on. Hundreds of surplus calories can be eaten this way, likely to contain little in the way of good nutrition. I also feel self-choice school lunches for children are a bad idea, as most will pick the fattiest, most calorific things. Lunch packed by you is a safer alternative and the only way to know what's being eaten.

One way to monitor your child's calorie intake is to revive family mealtimes. 'Proper' meals have mostly been replaced by eating on the hoof or in front of the TV. If you don't want your child to be overweight, you need to take back control of what he/she eats and drinks and how much exercise he/she does. Children are too young to know what's best for them, or care about their health. Given the choice, most will pick snack foods high in fat, salt and/or sugar rather than fresh fruits, salads, etc. If allowed to get into the habit, they'll also prefer to sit and be entertained than get out and be active. Too much freedom to choose their own diet and too many hours in front of the TV/computer will make a very high percentage of them fat.

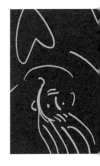

for kids (and parents) only

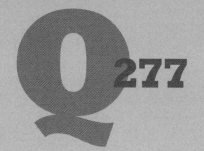

Q 277 Is it true that you should never put a child on a low-calorie diet?

Although many experts say you shouldn't put overweight children 'on a diet', as we've seen, very many children DO need to lose weight – so it's catch-22 – if you can't put your child on a diet, how is he/she ever going to lose weight? Calorie restriction seems to me to be an almost essential part of the equation.

Here we have the dilemma of what a 'low-calorie diet' means. If you give your child a healthy diet with restricted fat and restricted sugar but with extra fruit and vegetables and bread, for example, so that the total calorie content is reduced but he/she still has plenty to eat, that's a reduced-calorie diet. But perhaps a low-calorie diet conjures up meagre rations of lettuce and cottage cheese. So if 'low-calorie' in your book equates with 'crash dieting' then certainly don't put your child on one of those.

This isn't only because it will be demoralizing and miserable for them, but also because all children need all the nutrients necessary to grow and build bone, muscle, organs, etc. They also need all the vitamins and minerals to help this along and ensure health. A poorly thought-out calorie-reduced diet, especially one too low in calories overall, may not supply all these.

It's fair to say that any parent who feels their child is overweight should first see a doctor (who may refer you to a dietitian) and follow their guidelines. Having said that, obviously if your child's been eating lots of sweet snacks, crisps, etc. no dietitian is going to say you can't try to cut these out, or down. Often such methods will be enough in themselves to help a child slim over time and this is dieting by any other name.

I suppose the key is that children should be helped to lose weight, if necessary, in a gradual, non-obtrusive way that won't have them feeling hungry or rebellious, or make them feel 'at fault' or depressed with their weight. Some experts believe the best way to slim down a fat child is simply to try to maintain his/her weight at its current level and wait until he/she literally 'grows into' it. You still need to watch the calories, but looking at this long-term picture may be better for the child psychologically and physically. You never once need say to the child 'you have to lose weight' and he/she can follow a 'calorie-containing' diet rather than a 'calorie-restricted' diet, so it may make him/her feel better all round. Just check his/her weight from time to time, and if he/she hasn't put on any more, all is well.

Again, the doctor/dietitian who knows the child may offer the best advice on which method to follow. All the advice on feeding overweight children in the rest of this section is general, but it is always wise to treat your child as an individual.

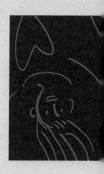

for kids (and parents) only

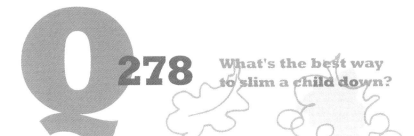

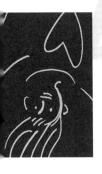

The previous questions will tell you broadly the lines along which to think. Here are more detailed guidelines:
• Aim at a weekly weight loss of up to $^{1}/_{2}$-1lb (225–450g), meaning reducing daily calorie intake by about 250–500, which isn't drastic and should ensure adequate nutrition.
• If your child has been having regular snacks of sweets, biscuits, crisps, etc. and a lot of high-sugar drinks, these are the first things to cut right back on, replacing them with less energy-dense foods such as those suggested in Questions 285–7. For some children, this alone is enough to produce 1lb a week loss.
• Limit takeaway meals and meals eaten outside your control – prepare food yourself where possible.
• Don't reward good behaviour with snacks or chocolates and aim gradually to alter his/her mindset into accepting that food isn't always associated with 'leisure and pleasure': for example, a visit to the cinema needn't mean a huge box of popcorn.
• An easy method for both parent and child to follow is the 'Traffic Light' system in Question 95.

Q279

Should I take my overweight child to the doctor?

In theory, it's always best to visit the doctor, but in practice things don't always go that smoothly, particularly if the child has low self-esteem. Having your size discussed by adults is quite demoralizing, and it can backfire, with the child becoming uncooperative or depressed.

It's best to help a child slim without him/her quite realizing what's going on – possible if you go for very slow weight loss. Yet I feel the doctor visit is the right way to go. You could explain the problem to the doctor beforehand and he/she might help invent another reason for the visit – e.g. a general check-up. There is then naturally a weigh-in and the subject of weight control can be gently introduced. Some doctors are excellent at this.

Otherwise, if the problem seems minor and you think you can beat it simply by altering snacking habits, then perhaps you can manage without a visit. What you don't want to do is give any child a complex about his/her weight. Encourage, or even slightly cajole, but never bully them about their weight/diet. Question 298 discusses the psychology of slimming for the young.

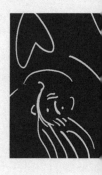

for kids (and parents) only

357

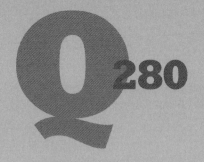

Q280 How can I stop my child aged 7 from liking junk food like burgers, which will no doubt make him fat eventually?

The occasional lean burger won't make your child fat if it's part of a healthy balanced diet. Nutritionally, they aren't all bad, containing good amounts of iron, B vitamins and protein, and calcium in the bun. For more on 'junk' food and takeaways, see Questions 100, 125 and 150. You'll see that there are reasonable fast-food choices. Remember, though, that most such food is also high in salt and some made from low-quality meat.

If your child is pre-teen, they don't need as many calories as a teenager, and neither should they get so much fat. So, if regularly having adult portions, they're probably getting more of both than needed and will gain weight. For example, your seven-year-old needs a maximum of about 76g of fat a day and 1,970 calories. An average (small) cheeseburger in a bun with fries and a regular milkshake contains about 1,150 calories and 44g fat. So one meal provides over 58% of daily calorie needs and 58% of fat allowance. The rest of the day's meals need to be lower in fat and calories – and contain fruit and veg – to give a balanced diet that won't put weight on.

The first thing to do, if serving your child burgers, pizzas, nuggets, etc. at home, is to reduce portion sizes and offer veg, salad and fruit with them. The second is to restrict these meals to a few times a week – perhaps reducing gradually over time. The third thing to do is to drum up a repertoire of alternative meals to which they won't object. There are several ideas throughout this section, and elsewhere in the book. If any child has a normal appetite and you continue to present them with meals other than the one or two favourites (without making a big deal of it), they usually capitulate through hunger and end up enjoying the food in question. I know that none of this will be easy, but just be quietly determined.

One compromise might be to cook homemade 'junk'! For example, burgers made from lean mince, pizzas with more tomato and less fatty topping, and so on. Also, encourage your child to exercise to burn off surplus calories before they turn into fat.

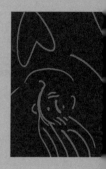

The best way to help your child to long-term health and weight control is to introduce a wide variety of foods, including fresh fruits, veg and salads, from toddlerhood and to rely on convenience foods as little as possible. The taste for salty, sugary and fatty foods is learnt early, and it is a lot easier to prevent them getting the habit than to cure it once it has taken hold!

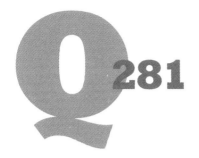

Q281

My son has a huge appetite and is putting on weight, yet if I cut portions he gets very hungry. What can I do?

First check that he really is overweight (Question 275) – if prepubescent, his increased appetite and weight may be natural. If really overweight, you need to cut his calorie intake a little, but rather than cut the portion in total, make sure the parts you reduce are those that are densest – highest in calories weight for weight. In general, these will be foods highest in fat.

For example, if you usually offer two large lamb chops, for example, but substitute two small well trimmed ones instead, you might save as much as 500–600 calories and 50–55g of fat. So that you still have a plate of food that looks plenty, what you do then is add extra of the lower-density, lower-fat, lower-calorie foods. For example, doubling the portion of peas would add only an extra 50 or so calories and increasing the portion of mashed potatoes by one-third would only add about 100 calories. You might have taken away 100g (3$\frac{1}{2}$oz) of food via the chops, but you've added 175g (6oz) of healthy veg losing a net total of over 400 calories in the process.

It is remarkably easy in this way to offer a large plateful of food while reducing the calories on the plate considerably. The 'Traffic Light' system explained in Question 95 is also good to follow, as you don't even have to worry too much about portion sizes – he/she can 'eat all they want' of the 'Green for go' foods. You can apply the same calorie-reducing principles to puddings, too, and in fact any meal at all. The final thing to do is bulk up the plate even more with low-calorie salads and veg.

Other points to note about appetite appear in Question 20. It is especially important with hungry children who may be getting overweight to try to slow down their rate of eating and get them to concentrate more on the taste, texture and enjoyment of food. It is better for children to eat at a table with the family and chat during the meal – the rate of eating will naturally slow down then. Food gulped down mindlessly while watching TV gets eaten at twice the rate and the child is likely to ask for seconds, as his/her appetite mechanism won't have time to register being full.

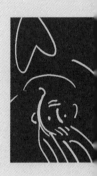

It is also a good idea to ensure a child doesn't go for too long without anything to eat. I am all for between-meal snacks if healthy – a 100-calorie snack of a slice of bread with low-fat spread and Marmite will take the edge off appetite at hungry times (say, on getting in from school) so at mealtime he/she won't be so ravenous.

Q 282

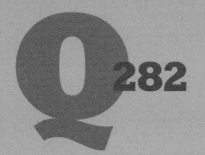

Is it OK to reduce fat in children's diets or do they need more than adults?

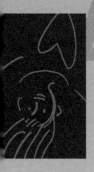

From weaning to about 5, children do need more fat. Amounts recommended for children reflect a gradual cutting down of fat intake from 42% at age 1 to 35% at 5. From 1 to 2, give them whole milk, from 3 to 5 semi-skimmed can be given, but fully skimmed milk not until after 5. Remember that, although children need more fat, it's best as part of decent-quality food, like full-fat cheeses, rather than 'junk'.

By school age, children don't really need more fat – consider 35% of calories plenty. Ensure it's mostly unsaturated, and that it includes plenty of the healthy-fat foods, such as oily fish, nuts, seeds and good-quality plant oils. Cut right back on saturated fats in items such as cream, cream cheese, fatty meats, pastry, cakes, biscuits, etc.

There's no need to cut out the medium-fat saturated fat foods such as most cheeses, eggs, milk and lean meats that provide a range of minerals and vitamins important for growth and health. Low-fat foods like low-fat cheeses, low-fat yoghurt and skinless poultry are useful. For more on fats, see Question 72.

Q283 If my child is overweight is fat the first thing to restrict?

See the previous question. Most experts suggest the first things to restrict are low-nutrient 'junk' foods and drinks, which offer little nutrition but are high in calories. Some, but not all, will be high in fat, others high in sugar, some in both. Next think about cutting out sweets and chocolates, then snacks like crisps. Also consider cutting high-fat, sugary puddings and savoury pastries like sausage rolls. These are all generally the first things to restrict and for many children will be enough to instigate weight loss.

Q284 Is a high-fibre diet suitable for all children?

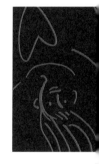

Very small children shouldn't be given a lot of very-high-fibre foods, as their systems won't cope and mineral absorption may be hindered. Young slim children with small appetites find high-fibre foods daunting as they need lots of chewing and make them full before getting many calories – why they're good for older overweight children. Foods like wholewheat pasta and pulses should feature in their calorie-controlled diet unless there are medical reasons not to (check with the dietitian).

for kids (and parents) only

Q285

How can I avoid my child eating sweets when she starts school?

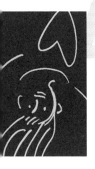

If a child hasn't been allowed sweets it's inevitable she will be offered them when she begins to mix with other children, and she will accept as it's natural for children to be curious about something which a) obviously everybody enjoys and b) has for her been banned. One study found children whose parents forbade them sweets and fizzy drinks were more likely to have them in secret.

So she will try sweets. All you can do is impress on her that sweets eaten between meals are not good for her teeth, and avoid buying them. Pester power becomes very strong once children start school, though, so be prepared for some battles.

Eventually you may decide it's best to limit sweets to a few after a meal, after which she cleans her teeth... a compromise. You can also choose the slightly 'better' sweets, such as good-quality chocolate or liquorice, rather than those that are pure sugar and spend a long time in the mouth. You may also cut back on sugar in other forms in her diet – for example, by avoiding over-sweet commercial cakes, biscuits and desserts.

Q286

What's the best way with a child's high intake of sweets and chocolate – banning or using as occasional treats?

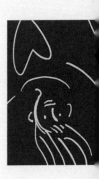

Once children reach school age, it's hard to police a complete ban on sweets and chocolate – they'll always find some, more so if you disapprove. Banning gives children a sweet tooth almost as much as giving treats and rewarding good behaviour with sweets because the child comes to think that if something is so good it's widely available and yet so bad you don't want them to have even one occasionally, it's got to be worth trying – and lying – for.

So I wouldn't ban them, but neither would I use them as occasional 'treats'. Tell your children sweets are 'empty' calories with virtually no nutrients, they're high in calories and may make them fat, they can contribute to tooth decay and may contain lots of unhealthy additives. Tell them if they would like to try a pack now and then, bought out of their pocket money with your knowledge, then that's up to them, but you think it's a waste of money.

Try to instil in children that a real sweet treat would be something like a bowlful of summer strawberries, or homemade bread with some local honey.

for kids (and parents) only

365

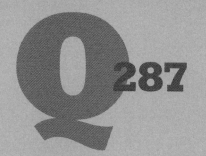

Q287

Any ideas for healthy, less fattening alternatives to sweets and crisps?

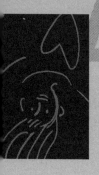

Dried fruits like sultanas and apricots are ideal (they're quite high in calories, but less so than sweets, and contain a good range of nutrients and fibre). Obviously, fresh fruit is a good choice. Lots of children don't like 'hard-to-eat-or-peel' fruits, such as oranges and grapefruit, and find apples hard to bite into. The fruits I find children most willing to eat are berries like strawberries, bananas, kiwi fruit, seedless satsumas and seedless grapes.

If it must be something less obviously healthy, then there are some sweets that are better for them – good-quality liquorice and chocolate aren't bad, and organic muesli bars are reasonable (though high in sugars).

As an alternative to crisps, you can get lower-salt, lower-fat crisps, and health-food shops stock organic crisps, also often lower in salt and fat. I recommend fresh nuts for children over 5 who aren't allergic – they're not low in calories, but contain essential fats shown to help children to health and brainpower. Avoid walnuts as most kids find them too bitter. Over-5-year-olds may also like two of my kid's favourites – pumpkin seeds and pine nuts.

Q288

You could be 'dieting' him on too few calories, so he's hungry – hence bad-tempered. He could be suffering 'withdrawal symptoms' from sweet or salty foods – try the suggestions in Question 133. It could be he feels isolated (especially if you've other children eating differently from him – see next question).

At 10 he's old enough to explain his feelings – so encourage him to voice his concerns and see if you can resolve them. Explain why he needs to watch his weight and suggest nice reasons for doing so – e.g. new clothes, etc. You must break the pattern of tantrums; he's hoping if he makes life difficult enough, you'll succumb.

Take him to your GP, who will reinforce the message if necessary. If your child receives instructions from an outsider he may feel more like complying. Some slimming clubs also allow children in and have a good success rate.

If you can offer him satisfying meals containing at least mostly foods he doesn't dislike, and if you can motivate him, things should improve. As soon as he begins to look slimmer, his attitude will improve.

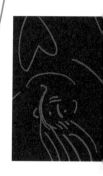

for kids (and parents) only

Q289

I have 3 children, but only one boy is overweight, causing endless problems at mealtimes and the overweight child feels bad. Any solutions?

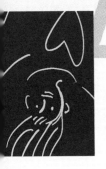

Feed the whole family a good healthy diet and simply give your overweight child slightly smaller portions, especially of high-density, high-fat foods, such as butter, cheese, etc. but give him extra veg to fill his plate. You can cut calories surreptitiously, a little here and there, to help him lose weight slowly. If the basic meal is the same as everyone else's, he'll probably be fine with reduced-fat, reduced-sugar products elsewhere.

If he has packed lunches, use this opportunity to reduce fat content (see Question 295). It would be best if they all have healthy desserts, rather than high-sugar, high-fat ones. If the slim children are still hungry, they can fill up on bread and honey or similar. Alternatively, they could have full-fat cream on their fruit, for instance, while he has 8%-fat fromage frais, which tastes nice.

Try to limit occasions when the other children tuck into pizza and he can't – of course he'll feel he's missing out. Make your own lower-fat pizza and let him tuck in too. I'm sure the answer mostly lies in 'portion control' and saving a few calories here and there.

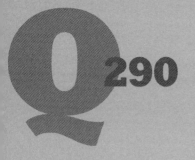

Q 290

Can you give me ideas for main meals for overweight children who only really like burgers, chips and baked beans?

Work new foods into their diet over the months. Borrow ideas from the retraining framework in Question 133, and a look at some of the rest of this section will give you ideas too (e.g. Questions 278, 280, 281 and 292).

However, a healthy eating diet and a weight-loss diet aren't the same. If your children are overweight, they could theoretically lose weight even while still eating burgers, chips and beans. You would simply have to cook the meal in the lowest-fat, lowest-cal way possible, i.e. extra-lean burger, large-cut oven chips or home-made potato wedges, and plenty of baked beans (low in fat and calories), but avoid giving too many chips, and make sure the rest of the day's food is not too high in calories and fat either.

As I've said, a lot of the foods we regard as 'junk' do, in fact, have good points. You may just need to do some 'tweaking' to make their food intake both healthy and non-fattening. For overweight children it's best to start by cutting sugary drinks, fatty/sugary desserts and similar snacks.

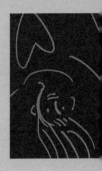

for kids (and parents) only

369

Q291

My 12-year-old always picks the most fattening/unhealthy items; how can I persuade him to healthier choices?

I can think of examples of the kind of situation you mean – the school café, where he goes for sausage and chips rather than chicken salad; the morning out with friends in town, when he goes to the burger bar; the pocket money spent on chocolate and sweets; the hand in the biscuit tin rather than the fruit bowl when he gets home from school.

I have had one such boy myself and I can tell you two things. One, it's hard, as they get older and start having a life and money of their own, to control what foods and snacks they buy, so it's best to try to give them a taste for decent food before they get into double figures, and to talk to them about what makes a healthy diet, and why. When all around him are eating rubbish, he's not likely to pick salad and water, so you have to be realistic. Maybe we should encourage our children to be friends with the ones who like healthy food, as well as those who don't swear and say 'please' and 'thank you'! We should also encourage our children not to be afraid to be individual – to lead rather than follow.

Two, you have to exert what influence you can and feel sure it will make a difference to the overall calorie content and nutritional quality of his diet. For example, you could make sure that at least at home there are no fizzy drinks and biscuits, and that whatever meals you give him are fairly low in fat and sugar, and not too calorific.

You could also go down the vanity route, and tell him that a healthy diet will give him better skin, more admiration from the girls, etc. I don't see any point, though, in turning yourself into the diet police – this will just antagonize him and make him eat all the more of everything you despise.

Lastly, remember that if he isn't overweight he can actually eat more food than you as he goes through his teens – from 15 to 18, boys have higher calorie needs than any other group – and that most food does have some nutrients in it. If he looks as if he's starting to put on weight, be extra-vigilant about not offering sugary drinks and high-fat, high-sugar things at home, and encourage him to take more exercise.

With regard to school meals, in the UK new rules insist that school canteens are required to meet certain nutritional standards, for instance offering fish at least twice a week and fruit and veg every day. This still leaves the problem of choice, and chips are on the menu for over-11s every day. But at least it's an improvement.

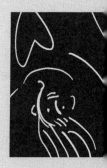

for kids (and parents) only

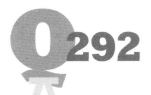

Q292

How do I give my kids reduced-fat/cal food so they don't realize?

Say 'diet' to most children and they get uncooperative. It's best simply to provide them with reduced-cal meals without making an issue of it. Don't mention words like 'low-calorie' or 'can't have'. The trick is to think of plenty of tasty things they can have and couple that with slight portion control to get the desired effect over time. There is no hurry and, as we saw in Question 277, you could even simply keep them at their current weight so they grow into it. Also, the more exercise they do, the more they can eat.

Q293

What is the best exercise for an exercise-shy child?

This depends on the reason for the dislike. If they find it boring, dress it up to seem like fun – making a walk into a treasure hunt, etc. If he/she finds it difficult, then develop confidence with family activities like cycling or swimming. Encourage rather than bully and avoid situations where he/she is forced to exercise with children he/she doesn't know well. Perhaps the best solution is to begin a 'walk to school' regime. Most children persuaded into exercise seem quite quickly to find they actually enjoy it.

Q 294

It's a good idea for all children to start the day with a breakfast. Research shows it improves concentration and brainpower in the morning. If they skip it, as with adults, their blood sugar levels will be low until lunchtime. A good breakfast should contain plenty of fast- and slow-release carbs (see Question 66), such as bread, cereal, porridge, bananas and dried fruit, for instant and more sustaining energy, as well as some protein (milk, yoghurt, baked beans, egg), a little fat (the spread on the bread, milk, yoghurt, nuts and seeds) and something to provide vitamin C (e.g. fresh fruit or fruit juice).

If the child enjoys a hearty breakfast, he/she could have a bowl of cereal with milk and chopped fruit, followed by a slice of bread with spread and some low-sugar jam or marmalade, otherwise skip the bread. If the child doesn't like breakfast, you could simply make a milkshake by blending semi-skimmed milk, banana, berry fruits and honey. Adjust the size of the packed lunch according to how much breakfast your child prefers to eat.

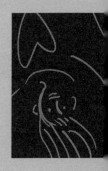

for kids (and parents) only

Q295 Can you advise me on healthy low-cal packed lunches for my children?

A good basic packed lunch will contain a carbohydrate element, a protein element, some fresh fruit and/or vegetables, something semi-sweet, and a drink. None of these are high in calories or fat:

CARBS: brown, white, wholemeal or rye bread, rolls, bagel, pitta, cooked rice, couscous or pasta.

PROTEIN: medium- or low-fat cheeses, such as Edam, half-fat Cheddar, egg, extra-lean ham, breast of chicken, turkey, prawns, tuna canned in brine, tinned pink salmon. Any fruits and vegetables.

SEMI-SWEET ITEMS: malt loaf, homemade fruitcake, tea bread (e.g. date and nut, bara brith), digestive biscuits.

DRINKS: water, diluted fruit juice, semi-skimmed milk (or homemade milkshake with blended fresh fruit).

For a slightly hungrier child you could add an extra or two – e.g. some dried fruit, some fresh nuts (if he/she isn't allergic to them) or seeds, or some low-fat, low-salt crisps. To help keep the fat content of the lunch down for weight-watching children, use low-fat spread or low-cal mayo on the bread, rather than butter or full-fat margarine.

In winter, buy an individual-sized, wide-necked soup vacuum flask so the child can take a homemade soup to school with some bread, instead of the sandwich. In summer, you can use leftover cooked brown or white rice, couscous or pasta shapes to make a salad which he/she can take to school in a lidded plastic container, with a plastic spoon and fork, again instead of the sandwich. The advantage of soups and salads is that you can work in fresh veg and salad items in greater quantities than you can get inside a sandwich – and in my experience, a lot of children won't eat salad items inside bread, in any case.

A moderate-calorie lunch for an average child should contain around 500–600 calories and all the following examples contain around that.

• Sandwich with half-fat Cheddar and pickle; 1 satsuma, 1 small banana, 1 slice of malt loaf; diluted apple juice.
• Soft brown bap filled with cooked chicken breast and crisp lettuce with low-fat mayonnaise; 3 whole cherry tomatoes; 1 slice of tea bread; 1 small bag of raisins and cashews (not for nut allergy sufferers); water.
• Leftover cooked brown rice mixed with chopped cucumber, celery, nuts (not for nut allergy sufferers), apple and dried apricot, plus some chopped cooked chicken or cheese and French dressing (or whatever dressing the child will eat); 2 digestive biscuits; diluted orange juice.
• Leftover cooked pasta shapes mixed with chopped tomato, red onion, cucumber, cooked broccoli florets mixed with chopped mozzarella cheese and some mayonnaise thinned down with a little skimmed milk and seasoning; 1 satsuma; 1 slice of fruit cake; water.

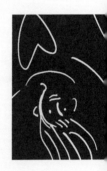

for kids (and parents) only

Q296

Is there such a thing as puppy fat and, if there is, will it go with age?

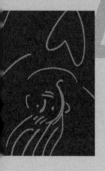

Physiological changes at adolescence predispose to increased fat deposition, especially in girls – the increased fat on the breasts, hips, bottom and thighs normal for the female. The laying down of surplus fat can trigger the onset of puberty, hence increased appetite.

These factors can make some children, especially girls, put on fat rapidly from 12 to 14. It's important to establish whether this is within the normal range for their age and height, perhaps with a doctor's help. Obviously, when a girl gets curves this shouldn't be confused with overweight. A good indication is if her waist is still well defined, then she's probably not overweight.

Adolescent weight gain, it's often said, will naturally disappear. If a child has had a sharp increase of appetite around puberty, sometimes this naturally decreases. However, in many cases, this doesn't happen and the child continues to put on weight and may get fat. However, most adolescents are several inches taller by the time they're fully grown, so the 'wait for extra height' policy in Question 277 may work for all but the most obese.

Q 297

Are any forms of exercise dangerous for a child?

A

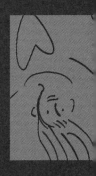

Some professionals feel it isn't a good idea for very young children to perform resistance exercise, as bones and bodies are growing rapidly and such exercise could cause injury, etc. In the US, however, the Kid's Activity Pyramid – guidelines used by health professionals, teachers, etc. – suggests regular muscle-strengthening exercise is important for all children, as it not only helps build physique and burn calories, but can also reduce the risk of osteoporosis later. They say weight-bearing exercise can be carried out, as long as weights are moderate and muscle strength is increased by additional repetitions.

What the American Academy of Pediatrics say shouldn't be attempted until growth is completed are lifting heavy weights, power-lifting, bodybuilding and repetitive use of very heavy weights. Most girls don't finish growing until 16, boys until 18. The AAP also say young children may not be suitable for distance running or intensive training as there may be musculo-skeletal and other damage. Their message is that any child participating in such activities should be monitored by a health professional.

for kids (and parents) only

Q298 How does one stop a child from getting obsessive about dieting?

Research seems to show that young girls (and boys to a lesser degree) are largely influenced in attitude to food, their bodies and 'diets' by their mothers' (and sometimes fathers') attitudes. Eating disorder centres see children as young as 8 and even 3- and 4-year-olds can be made over-anxious and conscious of food by parents' attitudes. Glasgow Royal Hospital for Children has found that, ironically, parents over-anxious to give their children a healthy diet, and for them not to be overweight, may in fact encourage eating problems. Over-strict parents who ban a range of perceived 'unhealthy' or 'fattening' foods are, they believe, inviting problems with eating disorders or, conversely, encouraging obesity by having the opposite effect to that intended. (If you can't have something, you may want it all the more.)

In particular, parents who are obsessive slimmers or health-food fanatics may find their children are more inclined to diet, be figure-conscious and have a poor self-image than others even when not overweight. A mother's worries about her figure and diet are particularly likely to be emulated by her daughter, according to a Boston study. Another found daughters whose appearance had been criticized by mothers were more likely to diet and 'yo-yo'.

So what to do? Obesity is a major anxiety, and so a real weight problem in a child shouldn't be ignored. BUT the idea of eating as a pleasant, relaxed event and food as an enjoyable part of living should be encouraged and overemphasis on calorie-counting be avoided.

Equally important is that the parents should show a similarly relaxed attitude – eating well and healthily, but not being obsessive about food, diets, etc. They should be comfortable in their own bodies, taking adequate (not obsessive) exercise, and a not unhealthy interest in their appearance. In other words, moderation is the key.

Be a good role model and, hopefully, your children will not become obsessive or suffer eating disorders. Your attitude until they're around 12 is the most important. After that, peer pressure to be slim, etc. may play an equally important role in how your child views her/his body and eating habits. At this time you need to carry on with the same 'good role model' philosophy and keep a discreet eye on your child's feelings on the subject, while being as positive as possible regarding their appearance.

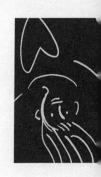

It's also worth noting that many anorexics and bulimics come from homes where very high standards of academic achievement are expected. If you feel you may be inclined to expect too much of your child, try to moderate that too.

A survey by the Schools Education Unit showed over half of all girls aged 12–15 wanted to lose weight, though most weren't clinically overweight.

for kids (and parents) only

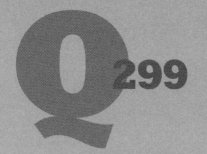

Q299 What are the signs of anorexia or bulimia in a teenager?

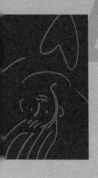

The signs may be similar to those for adults (see Questions 135 and 137). An anorexic or pre-anorexic teenager might refuse to eat with the family and lie about what food she/he has eaten or talk about food and dieting a lot – one survey reveals that dieting is the strongest indicator of eating disorders. Meals may be skipped – particularly breakfast and lunch at school. She/he may try to disguise a thin body with layers or baggy clothes; may seem withdrawn and may also do a lot of exercise.

Many teenagers with eating disorders become obsessive about food – cooking food for you, taking cookery lessons at school and even wanting a career in catering. Bulimics may lie or steal to get money for food, or steal food. Both potential anorexics and bulimics may be over-anxious, often about schoolwork or performance, and have high standards.

It's estimated that up to 10% of teenagers have a 'pre-anorexic' mild eating disorder, when they skip meals and are thinner than is healthy, while saying they're fat. At this stage, with care, the problem is easier to solve.

Q 300

What should I do if I think my child may have an eating disorder?

If you suspect a child has an eating disorder, do what you can to discover the truth – many children will deny there is a problem, but a talk with the school or college head, or even with worried friends, may bring the problem to the surface. Although teenagers do talk a lot about diets, body image and so on, when a friend actually succumbs to an eating disorder they are understandably worried and may be relieved to confide in an adult.

Do take your child to the doctor if you suspect an eating disorder. You can also contact one of the help lines given in Question 134 and you'll be offered counselling for the child or whole family, as well as medical help. Eating disorders are notoriously difficult to self-treat and unlikely to go without professional help.

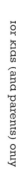

Index (see also the list of questions on pages 4–9)

abdominoplasties 53, 80
acupuncture 182
aerobics 17, 47, 59, 74, 273, 275, 277, 285, 287-8, 294
ageing and weight 25, 33, 40-1, 336-7, 339-41
alcohol 85-6, 89, 138, 213, 226-7, 269, 313, 343, 345, 347
Alexander Technique 69, 81
allergies, food 140-1, 142-3
anorexia 186-7, 188, 189, 192, 379, 380
appetite 27, 36-7, 176, 274-5, 340, 360-1
    suppressants 37, 50, 55
apple shape 39, 73, 74, 98, 244-5, 266, 268, 344, 345
aromatherapy 182
arthritis 23, 264-5, 337
Atkins Diet 125
Ayurveda 182

bad breath 88, 105
basal metabolic rate 14, 15, 17, 24, 27, 34, 35, 38
binge eating 90, 94, 116, 186, 193
bloating 140-1, 308
    see also fluid retention
blood pressure, high 73, 75, 110, 111, 241, 245, 254, 263, 273
blood-sugar levels 16, 37, 101, 115, 116, 117, 147, 178, 205, 229, 256-7, 258, 304
BMI see Body Mass Index
BMR see basal metabolic rate

body fat 12, 14, 27, 41, 42, 46, 49, 316
Body Mass Index 42, 44-5, 58, 240, 242, 243, 247, 268
bones 12, 44, 88; see also osteoporosis
books 183
bottoms 66, 68, 69, 70;
breakfasts 117, 185, 208, 211, 233, 373
breasts 61, 63, 76, 314, 316
    flabby (men) 347
budget eating 230-4
bulimia 186, 187, 190-1, 192, 379, 380

caffeine 19, 120, 121, 172
calories 14, 15, 31, 32, 50, 52, 84, 85, 89, 123, 124, 126-7, 130, 135, 151, 248
cancers 23, 111, 240-1, 337
carbohydrates 51, 52, 58, 85, 86, 89, 90-1, 96-7, 100, 134, 137, 166-7, 222, 223, 232, 262, 289
cellulite 318, 319, 320
cheese 107, 138, 139, 149, 224, 237
children 307, 350-81
chocolate 19, 107, 138, 147, 167, 171, 172-3, 310
cholesterol 73, 91, 108, 109, 110, 111, 241, 254, 267, 269
clubs, slimming 155, 169, 183, 271, 367
coaches, diet 183
coffee 19, 172, 313, 315
constipation 28, 88, 97, 105, 308

convenience food 194-5, 202-3
cooking 150, 200, 228
counselling 167, 168, 182
crash diets 47, 48, 49, 51, 58, 128, 189, 253
cravings 147, 167, 178, 310-11, 328

dairy produce 139, 140, 235, 236, 237
death, overweight and 39, 41, 42, 45, 244-5
depression 23, 33, 94, 166, 167, 182, 255, 309;
    see also SAD
desserts 148, 221, 223-4
'detox' diets 260-2, 318
diabetes/diabetics 73, 93, 95, 98, 240-1, 245, 254, 256, 258-9, 266, 267
dietary induced thermogenesis 14, 15, 17, 18, 22, 27, 35, 104-5, 133
diets, 'perfect' 122, 123
    most popular 124-5
dizziness 88, 101, 116
drinks 34, 120-1, 138, 185, 215, 275;
    see also alcohol, water
drugs: and weight gain 23, 33; see also pills

eating disorders 261, 271, 378-9, 381;
    see also anorexia; etc
eating habits, changing 22, 134, 161, 162, 170, 175, 184-5

eating out 32, 212-3, 217-25
ectomorphs 64
EFAs *see* essential fatty
   acids
eggs 18, 105, 236
elimination diets 265
emotional factors 16, 168
endomorphs 65
endorphins 172, 173, 310
energy 14, 17, 31, 33, 38
   deficits 31, 48, 50, 110,
   251, 289
essential fatty acids 111,
   309; *see also* omega fats
exercise(s) 17, 22, 24, 33, 37,
   40-1, 47-51, 57, 59, 61, 63,
   66, 75, 81, 127, 135, 137,
   157, 163, 255, 270, 272-305
   for children 372, 377
   for men 348
   post-menopausal 338-9
   postnatal 330, 331
   and pregnancy 329

F-Plan, The 125
faces 63, 76, 77
fast food 145, 146, 151, 160-
   1, 175, 204-5, 358-9, 369
fasting 88, 129, 256
fat *see* body fat; fats, intra-
   abdominal
fats, dietary 85, 86, 87, 89,
   106-11, 145, 146, 252
fatty acids 86, 87;
   see essential fatty acids
feminism 180-81
fibre 96-7, 100, 125, 263,
   269, 363
fluid retention 13, 32, 38,
   91, 142, 314-15
food-combining 112, 137

genes/genetics 26-7, 57,
   60, 186-7
GI see Glycaemic Index
glands 28-9
glucose 86-9, 92, 98, 267
Glycaemic Index 89, 98-9,
   124
gyms 59, 66, 284, 295, 302

Hay, William: diet 112, 137
health and weight 45,
   240-3, 246-7, 272-3
healthy slimming 248-51
heart disease 13, 41, 73, 93,
   110, 111, 120, 173, 241, 243,
   254, 266-9, 277, 337, 343
herbal supplements 21, 37
herbs 21, 85, 121, 165, 182
high-carbohydrate diets
   51, 96-7
high-fibre diets 96-7, 125,
   363
high-protein diets 104-5,
   125, 137, 225
hips 61, 70, 71, 72, 241, 316
holidays, slimming for 78
honey 93
hormone replacement
   therapy (HRT) 333, 334,
   335, 338, 339
hormones 28-9, 40, 41, 61,
   240, 310, 313
hotel meals 213, 218-19
hunger 100, 102-3, 161,
   170, 171, 311, 312
hypnosis 182

illnesses 23, 25, 33, 73, 305;
see also cancers; etc
insulin 73, 92-3, 100, 107,
   178, 256, 257, 311, 315

intra-abdominal fat 63, 72,
   73, 241, 267
iodine deficiency 19, 28
iron, dietary 235, 236, 237

ketones/ketosis 88, 105

lean tissue 41, 46, 47, 48,
   49, 58
liposuction 50, 53, 67, 70, 77
liquid-only diets 131, 253
low-carbohydrate diets
   223, 262
low-fat diets 51, 52, 58,
   110-11, 124-5, 137
lunches 101, 209, 211-2, 233
   packed 210, 214-15,
   229, 368, 374-5

massage 182
meal replacement diets 125
meals 22, 59, 116;
   see breakfasts etc
men 342-9
menopause 39, 334-5, 338-9
   male 349
mental activity 196
mesomorphs 62, 64-5
metabolism 18-19, 20-1, 47;
   see basal metabolic rate
minerals 86, 88, 121, 131, 139
motivation 154-5, 169, 176
muscles 12, 13, 46, 48, 58,
   62, 63, 299

'natural' weight 24, 34
'negative-calorie' foods 133
'night eating syndrome' 193
night workers 206-7
noradrenaline 29, 37, 310
nutrients 86, 88, 128, 235-6

obesity 12, 45, 163
oestrogen 310, 313, 314, 316, 318, 347
oils 85, 109, 252, 259, 264, 269
omega fats 107, 108-9, 111, 237, 252, 257, 261, 265, 269
orthorexia 188
osteoarthritis 264
osteoporosis 41, 243, 254, 268, 298, 336
Overeaters Anonymous 156, 168, 179
overeating 32, 168; see binge eating; bulimia
overweight 12, 42, 43, 45, 72, 159

patches, slimming 182
pear shape 61, 70-72, 266
phytochemicals 93, 269
Pilates 69, 75, 81
pills, slimming 21, 37, 50, 54-5, 132
'pinch test' 43
polyunsaturated fats 108-9
portion sizes 136
posture 66, 67, 68-9, 81
pregnancy 70, 271, 313, 316, 321-9
premenstrual problems 13, 36, 257, 308-15
proteins 18, 85, 86, 89, 99, 133, 232
psychological factors 16, 30, 38, 116, 153, 254-5, 257, 274
puppy fat 376

raw-food diets 113
ready meals 194-5, 202-3, 210

restaurants 213, 217, 223
rheumatoid arthritis 23, 264-5

salon wraps 67, 79
salt 149, 185, 263, 314, 315, 333
saturated fats 107, 108, 111
school meals 370, 371
seasonal affective disorder (SAD) 36-7, 166, 178
serotonin 37, 94, 166, 173, 178, 310
'set point' theory 24
sex 317
shiftworkers 206-7
skin folds, removing 53, 80
sleep 35, 118, 196
smoking 198, 199, 235, 245, 257
snacks 101, 115, 170, 171, 194, 195, 209, 210, 211, 216, 257, 311
spot-reduction 63, 71, 76
'starch-blockers' 132
step aerobics 286, 288
stomachs 67-9, 71, 75, 76, 81, 294, 346
strength training 298, 301
stress 16, 29, 182, 197, 257, 266
sugars 85, 86, 87, 89, 90, 92-3, 99, 184, 185, 229, 314-15
supplements 20-1, 37
surgery 50, 53, 67
sweeteners, artificial 94-5
sweets 364, 365, 366; see also chocolate; desserts
'Syndrome X' 337

takeaway meals see fast food
tea 19, 85, 120-1, 172, 269
teenagers 351, 371, 376, 379, 380, 381
thermogenesis see dietary thermogenesis
thighs 61, 70, 71, 72, 241, 316; see also cellulite
thyroid problems 19, 20, 23, 28, 29
tiredness 101, 116
toning exercises 63, 294
'traffic light system' 136, 138, 174, 225
trans fats 107, 108, 111
triglycerides 87, 269

vanilla 173, 182
vegetarians 235, 236-7, 265
vitamins 86, 88, 101, 131, 139, 203, 231, 236, 237, 264, 269, 309, 314, 315, 341
VLCDs 131, 253

waists 12, 42, 43, 45, 72, 73, 243
water 31, 37, 85, 120
weight 24-30, 42-5
gain 56-9, 163, 270; see also ageing
weight-training 294, 297
wheat products 140, 142-3
willpower 116, 161, 169

'yo-yo' dieting 48, 49, 128, 156, 242, 243, 254-5, 261, 263
yoga 62, 69, 75, 81, 182, 294, 301, 348
yoghurt 18-19, 98, 99